I'M GLAD YOU'RE NOT DEAD

To Claire,
With good
wishes for your
husband's health,
and your peace.

Sincerely,
Elizabeth Post

I'M GLAD YOU'RE NOT DEAD

A
LIVER TRANSPLANT
STORY

Elizabeth Parr

Published By

Journey Publishing
6610 Stewart Road, Suite 16
Galveston, Texas 77551

ISBN 0-9654728-0-9
Library of Congress Catalog Card Number: 96-094745

Journey Publishing
6610 Stewart Road, Suite 16
Galveston, Texas 77551

Printing by
D. Armstrong Book Printing Co., Inc.
Houston, Texas

Typography and Book Design by
Journey Publishing

Printed in the United States of America

Dedicated
to Natalie
and
to Janet.

Table of Contents

Table of Contents

Acknowledgments

Many persons, some immediate and some now remote, have contributed to my successful liver transplant, and hence to this book.

My mother and my father, Elizabeth and Rufus Parr, have supported me through many episodes in life, but heroically through this most traumatic one.

I am most grateful, too, for their support, to my immediate family, my sisters, Margaret and Kathy, and my brother, Dan.

To my immediate circle of friends, whose faces and love appeared when I most needed them: Catherine, Joan, Carol, Amy, Ellen, Emily, Sean, and Linda.

To my colleagues at the University of St. Thomas, but especially those who regularly checked on me, President Joe McFadden and Dr. Joy Linsley.

To those at the university and elsewhere who donated blood, sent cards, and said prayers.

Acknowledgments

To all of those who prayed for me, particularly those present and former Sisters of St. Mary, my colleagues in a timeless spiritual life.

To my surgeon, Thomas Broughan M.D., of the Department of Surgery at the University of Texas Medical Branch at Galveston, who not only saved my life through liver transplantation, but then patiently and kindly edited the medical terminology in this book. I acknowledge him gratefully for editing the contents of the glossary.

To my hepatologist, Natalie Murray M.D., formerly of UTMB and now on the faculty at UC Irvine, whose medical knowledge kept me alive until Tom Broughan could perform surgery. She, too, contributed to the accuracy of the technical material in this book, and shared her expertise in a taped interview.

To Janet Mize R.N., formerly the Liver Transplant Coordinator at UTMB, now occupying that role at UC Irvine. Janet kept me organized and vitalized during a fifteen month wait for a liver, and also supervised my lay attempts at being medically correct.

To the nurses and staff on 6B, in John Sealy Hospital at UTMB, so professional and so human, so kind and so competent.

Acknowledgments

To the members of the Liver Support Group at
UTMB, especially those who shared their own
experiences so generously in order to expand the
reach of this book.

To Ann, who provided my emotional support
during the long wait and the difficult aftermath. I
could not have survived or recovered without her.

A Liver Transplant Story

A Note to the Reader

Beginnings are always difficult. I am
dealing with two: the birth- gift of life which a liver
transplant affords, and the after beginning of a book
about the process. Perspective is a reach when one
is still standing smack dab in the middle of an
existential event. I hope a helpful objectivity is
attained for both the reader, and I, the author, in
this process of writing. I am reminded, as I
commence, of something a colleague of mine, a
playwright, once said: "I begin to write finally, when
it is easier to do so than not." This work is about the
process of liver transplantation, from an exploratory
and very personal point of view. It is also a
compendium of selected information about the total
process of liver transplantation, the agonizing wait,
the complex surgery, and the recovery period. This
book presents itself as an uncontrived frame

narrative, encompassing other case histories, technical information, and the attendant emotional and spiritual crises. I have been allowed, very generously, to draw from the experiences of my friends in our liver support group, as well as from the expertise of the medical team involved in liver transplantation at the University of Texas Medical Branch at Galveston, Texas.

I hope that this book contains the helpful information, now confirmed by experience, which I sought so desperately over a two year hiatus of living with a terminal liver disease, while waiting for a solution.

I hope even more that this work prompts those of you hesitating about organ donation to hesitate no longer, to sign a donor card, and inform a loved one of your decision. Then, don't leave home without it. In this book I tell it like it is--no politicizing and no half-truths. This is a true liver transplant story.

For the person who suspects or fears a liver disease, for the person facing transplant surgery, for desperately worried relatives and friends, I hope that this book accompanies you as the voice of a friend, on your journey, out of the darkness, into the light of self and health discovery. This is finally your book. Remember, I am still in process. This book really has no closure, just termination.

Chapter One
E. R.

On one of the last class days of the fall
semester, 1995, a freshman student of mine
approached me after class. He blurted out at me,
"I'm glad you're not dead!" Eighteen or nineteen, he
looked thirteen or fourteen, a "Generation X" kid,
kind of cuddly, a little weird, and very candid. I was
startled, and immediately interpreted his oblique
compliment as meaning class had gone well; he
hadn't been bored. He didn't mean that at all. He
explained that he had heard something about my
liver transplant, and so this was his sincere and
generous attempt at congratulations. He said that I
was a nice lady.

I'm glad I'm not dead, too, and that I am back,
happily coping with the Gregs of the world, being
kept young by their candor, and feeling very alive

3

in their presence. This is the story of how I got not dead.

My knowledge of a liver disease began in trauma, and with a call to 911. During the night of March 5-6, 1992, I vomited blood. This jarring episode occurred in my home, over the course of several hours. I threw up varying amounts of blood over night. I really do not know what I was thinking that I did not immediately alert my friend with whom I live and head for an emergency room. At age 55 I had never been sick. I had never been hospitalized, and like too many Americans, took my health for granted; like too many Texans I had an attitude of invulnerability. I blame our expansive horizons, chauvinism and bravado for this attitude, one which suited me to a tee. On the surface I present a persona of control. I am, for heaven's sake, a teacher. I have a professional image to uphold. My mother named me Elizabeth after the little British Princess. I could not be sick. I could not be having an emergency. It would go away. I considered Ann. She needed her sleep. She, too, was a teacher, and in her Kentucky bred stoicism, met crisis head on, but she taught an at-risk population of high school students, and was a dedicated and compulsive workaholic, a personality

4

facet which students and administrators exploited.
She should not be awakened in the middle of a school
night. Instead, and to what end, I do not know, I
dutifully and compulsively sponged up splattered
blood from around the commode with disposable
paper -- TP, tissue. After each upheaval I washed
my face and rinsed out my mouth as if I were
returning to a cocktail party rather than to bed. I
waited, not resting, until the blood filled my stomach
cavity enough to make me nauseous again,
sometimes a matter of two hours, and then repeated
my bathroom trip. As I grew weaker, and probably
less focused and deliberate, I did a not so impeccable
a job of sponging. Blood was spattered everywhere.
I remember holding on to the belief that it would
stop, and that in the morning I would decide what
was to be done. I prayed; I worried. As long as I still
moved and thought, I did not think that I could be
dying. Descartes was alive and well.

When I finally acknowledged that the
hemorrhaging was not going to just go away, and the
hour seemed appropriate, I awakened Ann and
suggested, in a deceptively calm manner that maybe
she had better take me to the hospital.

By this time I was exceedingly weak from loss
of blood and welcomed her sensible suggestion that
we call an ambulance because that way we would get

immediate attention at the emergency room. When the ambulance arrived, I walked to it, simply out of a ridiculous concern that the neighbors not see a stretcher. Ann followed in her car. Her actions during this initial trauma characterized her and her prudent, decisive and loving care throughout what was to become a very long ordeal. She is my best friend. A few years younger than I, Ann and I had already shared a great deal together, outrageous camping trips, seaside crabbing fests, and trips to her mountain home where we "collected" folklore. Now we were to enter into a new phase of our relationship, a far more somber one, but one in which I could count on her in the hard times, too. Loyalty characterizes her; our affinity is amazing. We are both Leos, both have brown eyes and now grey hair, but out of an original natural brown. We resemble sisters more than I and my family sisters do. We do not have to speak to know what the other is thinking. On this occasion, however, she did not know what I was up to, or we would have been at the hospital hours earlier, at the first heave.

The surgeon on call in the emergency room at my HMO hospital in Houston, Texas performed an endoscopy and diagnosed an ulcer. Blood tests revealed a diseased liver. I was assured that, while the liver was damaged, probably it would regenerate, the enzyme levels would lower in time, and that there was sufficient liver function for life. I was advised to avoid toxic substances (alcohol, drugs, tobacco) and to observe good habits of nutrition.

I had observed, and so had my friends and family, some jaundice before this episode, accompanied by frequent blood vessel breaks in my eyes, and, known only to me, nausea. The liver was cirrhotic - a term which means scarred. The scarred tissue is more or less pervasive, depending on the extent of the damage, and is non-functional.

I was attended in the hospital by the internalist on call, who was a member of the HMO with whom my institution, and I, had insurance. I continued to see her regularly, while she and I waited for better enzyme results. They never came. Over a period of more than twelve months, I waited, my condition deteriorated, and I continued to work regularly in a high stress professional capacity. I saw a gastroenterologist only once, at her insistence. There was no appreciable follow-up with him, and no real interest demonstrated on his part. Meanwhile, I was prescribed diuretics for water retention, and continued with frequent but non-efficacious check-ups.

I'm Glad You're Not Dead

I consider this brief medical summary as a kind of topic statement which will be developed subsequently. Unfortunately, mine is not atypical of the treatment usually given many liver patients. The average gastroenterologist takes a hands-off approach, more often than not, in patients with hepatic pathology. I am afraid that the explanation for this apathy is, all too often, culpable ignorance or plain stupidity on this specialist's part. Misdiagnosis is a common experience for hepatic patients. I will return to case histories of this sort.

For myself, my treatment continued as no treatment. One year from my first hospitalization after hemorrhaging and receiving 5 units of blood, the hemorrhage reoccurred, this time not in my home and under the loving care of my close friend. This time, in fulfillment of my professional duties, I was waiting in a hotel room in Houston, Texas for a Chicago poet who was to conduct a reading/lecture at the university where I was chair of the English department. The poet was Gwendolyn Brooks. I was alone. I had been nauseated for at least a day, but self-diagnosed myself as having a 24-hour virus and was convinced in my usual compulsive manner that the show must go on. To that end, I had driven from my condo in Galveston, to my campus in

E. R.

Houston, literally swerving dizzily 50 miles down a busy and dangerous freeway, in order to hand over my car to two waiting students who would drive to Ft. Worth to meet and escort our guest to Houston.

Somehow, that day, I met my classes and taught them coherently, all the while feeling weaker and weaker. At the end of the work-day, my secretary drove me to the hotel where the students would later deliver the poet in order for me to make final arrangements for her stay. I had a wait of a few hours, so I checked into her room, intending to rest until her arrival. Checking in and approaching the elevator are the last scenes I remember. My next conscious moment found me in a familiar ICU of a Houston hospital. I was conscious; my brain was processing, but I could not speak. I had been comatose for some 28 hours. At this point I must rely on the information gained from others in order to recap the terrifying experience.

I had passed out on the bathroom floor of the hotel room after vomiting blood. Apparently I missed the toilet; there was blood all over the floor. I was not discovered for eight hours. The long interval between check-in and discovery is owing, I am told, to the visitor and students being told by the desk that someone was occupying that room, and so they placed Miss Brooks elsewhere. The door was never opened. I can only attribute this mix-up to a change in desk clerks, because upon registration, I had clearly identified myself as the person who had made the reservation and was there to greet the visiting lecturer. I had told Ann that I would be late that night, returning home about 10:00 pm. As the evening lengthened, she received an anxious call from the students who had expected to meet me and to return my car so that I could drive home. Their call triggered an attempt on my friend's part to reach me at any of several possible places: my office, my sister's, friends' homes, to no avail. Finally, my sister, Margaret, insisted that security in the hotel break in to the room. She listened in horror by phone to the security guard broadcasting to the front desk that: "We have an emergency here." Fortunately, Margaret remembered my doctor's name and the hospital. She called my home, and informed Ann of the situation. Both literally flew to the hospital, Ann with dog in tow because she had no place to leave him overnight, and no idea of what she might find. Even now I am deeply pained by the terrible anxiety I caused these two dear people.

I had not wanted to inform my parents of my illness, so as not to worry them. As the eldest child, I have assumed this position, self-imposed, since the

age of reason. This time, being comotose, I was
finally out of control. The attending physician was
proposing life support and offering little hope of my
regaining consciousness ever. Margaret decided
that, under the circumstances, she must let Mom
and Dad know, and so the circle of those desperately
worried, dear people extended, like a pebble thrown
in a pool; it devolved to other circles of siblings,
friends, and professional colleagues. It was known
that I was a sick woman, a condition which for some
reason of perverse pride, I wanted kept hidden, and
which really, I continued to deny. Even now, after a
successful transplant, I cringe when anyone reminds
me of how I looked "before," indicating they knew all
along a great deal more than I was admitting.

On the occasion of this crisis, I did awake,
began to put together my situation, at least enough
to recognize the ICU, and with Ann's help to glean
some information about what had happened. My
strongest memory of first consciousness, before I
could speak, was of a male nurse, a former military
paramedic, egotistical and abrasive, impatient with
my efforts to communicate. I was vulnerable and
confused, weak and helpless, but perfectly capable of
homicidal thoughts. I remembered with alarm the
intense scenario taking place that day, I thought, on
my campus, without my indispensable leadership.

I'm Glad You're Not Dead

When I could speak, I asked for a phone, and was told: "Lady - there are no phones [for the patients] in ICU!" I had barely been proclaimed mentally competent, and I was back in charge. When I learned that my parents were coming, I began manipulating so that I could be in a private room, and they would not have to see me in the ICU. The doctor could not believe that I was even conscious, much less coherent. I asked every orderly who passed through, the date and time, so that I could be ready for the standard *compis mentis* quiz. I prevailed. My parents greeted me with swollen lip and nose tube, but more or less myself . My sister's means of informing our parents, I had thought, left a little to be desired. She determined to drive to Fort Worth, while I was still comotose, enlisted the aid of our friend Linda, and left my bedside. She thought she should tell them in person that I might be dying. All the while, of course, I might have been dying. It seemed a strange time to make a ten-hour round trip. A telephone call might have been better, but she reasoned that since they knew nothing of my illness officially (wrong - my mother, in her infinite wisdom, has foreknowledge of everything), the shock would be too awesome over the phone lines. The reader might notice that, in this high tech age, communications do not come off too well in this

E. R.

narrative. My friend, Carol, a psychotherapist,
assures me that those who care the most often act
out in extreme ways in such a crisis and Margaret's
reaction was "classic." That she cared, I know.
Among the five children in my family I was the
eldest and Margaret was the second child. We were
close in age and in friendship. As children she had
followed me around rather adoringly for which, back
then, I could have brained her. In this incident,
with me out of control, she began to asert the big
sister role which had been denied her by birth
order. After all, her name was Margaret. She was
next in line to the throne. She was also wonderfully
attentive and miserably worried.

A few days and bad meals later, I was
discharged, and returned to work one week hence.
This not so well equipped hospital, had managed to
cleanse my system of the ammonia which the
diseased liver could not discharge from my blood. I
had passed out from an accumulation of toxins in my
brain. A bleed is a common occurrence, always life-
threatening, to those suffering from liver disease. I
will never know with certainty if I ever had an
ulcer, or gastritis, or if all along, as later a
competent hepatologist was to discover, the culprit
was solely portal hypertension, causing dilated veins
in the stomach.

I'm Glad You're Not Dead

I left the hospital with a more tentative prognosis, no formula for treatment, a prescription which lowered my diuretic dosage, and a nutrition program which called for a low sodium, low protein (20 grams per day) regimen. Transplant was mentioned in the hospital as an option to death, by a very young resident. His argument was sensible enough: in one year, my liver numbers remained unchanged; I was certainly no better. I had added, to my fickle physique, a herniated navel, owing to a water retaining belly. Now, "they" wanted me to lower the daily diuretic dose. My mistrust of scientists, carefully nourished in a strong humanities education, was rapidly attaining empirical justification.

So far, I had been docile. My role in aggressive treatment had been limited to eclectic homeopathic practices. Ann and I haunted health food and drug stores. We seized on anything that promised liver cleansing: herbal teas, lemon juice and raisins (marinating overnight), silimarin capsules, juice fasts, steam sweats. We juiced anything that would squeeze. Most of it tasted nasty (tolerable if you remembered the apple!) but, boy was it pure! Once I OD'd on wheat grass. This time the ready regurgitation was very green. Ann had loyally grown boxes of the stuff, only to have to pitch it. I couldn't even look at it. At her insistence, I began to search for alternative medical programs, no matter what the financial cost. I had been badly jerked around, at the cost of more than a year of treatment. I was not going to die. I had almost believed, up until this point, that I could recover - miraculously, not by prayer, but by will and ignorance, and absurdity. Now I faced transplant as perhaps the only resort. I had harbored the procedure previously as a kind of negative 1 out of 10 chance for recovery. I did not want to die in surgery. I also would not trust the health care system, which had so mismanaged me, to preside over my demise. In their hands, I felt certain of the outcome. Somewhere in here a sea change took place. I was determined to live. I cannot stress enough how important attitude is in the process, but I had to learn that strength of will, and a positive attitude is a tinkling cymbal, without medical expertise. And so I sought it. I sought it with the passion of a lover. I was transformed into a stalker, believing now that a transplant was my only hope, and that I would live, that it offered a cure, not a threat, that it was a solution to an increasingly frustrating problem.

I'm Glad You're Not Dead

It was summer, some four months after my last bleed, and a time for a healing rest, and a restless quest.

Chapter Two
"Searching for Mr. Goodbar:"
A Good Team is Hard to Find

Between the first and second hemorrhages,
Ann and I had moved from Houston to Galveston.
The move was motivated entirely by financial
exigencies, but was, as destiny would have it,
providential. In my desperate search for a doctor,
or doctors, who could help me, I began seeing, for
treatment, a young internalist who practiced out of
the same HMO as my former physicians, but closer to
my residence. She, at least, increased the diuretics,
recognized that the fluid buildup was relocating from
belly to lungs, and that my worsening cough was not
bronchitis, as my former internalist had discerned
by looking in my ears! This gal I trusted, but she
was not a specialist. She was, however, a graduate of
the University of Texas Medical Branch at Galveston-
my new home town.

I'm Glad You're Not Dead

Concurrently, with my visits to clinic, Ann and I began communicating, by long distance, with various liver support groups and organizations, notably the American Liver Foundation (ALF). We learned of the transplant programs and surgeons in Houston, Dallas, and a new program, only a year old, right under our noses, less than a mile from home, in Galveston, Texas - the University of Texas Medical Branch in Galveston (UTMB).

Ann called the program coordinator at UTMB, pretending to be me. I don't know where my head was at this point, whether stuck again in some denial hole, or escaping into a fiction of my own creation. More than a few times in this peculiar adventure we resembled Lucy and Ethel, or more appropriately, Cagney and Lacy. There were certainly enough bad guys out there, real or imagined, deserving our attention. Most of them belonged to a health care organization.

Janet Mize, R.N., Liver Transplant Coordinator at UTMB answered our desperate, shy call. Warm, dear, friendly, funny Janet explained the program, offered reassuring statistics concerning the percentage of successes which the chief liver transplant surgeon, Dr. Thomas Broughan, enjoyed, and made an appointment for "me" to be evaluated for transplant.

My only effective endeavor was to talk with my HMO internalist about referring me to UTMB. She, too, had learned of the nascent transplant program through an alumni newsletter, and was disposed to cooperate, not being committed herself to restricting patients, to their disadvantage, to one set of doctors. I am most grateful to this young, enlightened physician. Upon her referral, even though the copayment would be significantly higher, I would receive insurance benefits outside my healthcare network. At this point, I assume the voice of advisor, from the pinnacle of experience. Anyone with a liver disease must search for a hepatologist, or in the scarcity of that specialist, at least a board certified gastroenterologist whose fellowship included hepatology experience. A patient should settle for no less. In the case of the surgeon, the potential patient should ask about the percentages of successful and unsuccessful transplants, and the original place of the doctor's transplant training. This procedure is new enough that a handful of surgeons can trace their education in the field to a pioneer practitioner who has devised and developed the best procedures. With regard to the program at any given institution, it is incumbent to discern not

how many transplants were performed, but how
many successful ones, without retransplantation.
This last issue separates the quacks from the talents.
Shocking as it may seem, in so new a field, but with
grants and monies involved, hospital teams have
been known to perform liver transplants with
questionable organs, and surgically risky patients in
order to bump up their stats. These programs exist
by the beneficence of the state. The administrators
are not impressed by the numbers of candidates for
transplants, but by the actual numbers of
transplants performed.

UTMB offered a coherent program and a precise
screening process. The potential candidate is put
through a rigid and thorough series of tests aimed at
discerning the extent and nature of the disease and
the patient's prognosis for a successful transplant,
should one be in order. The team was composed in
1993 of the nurse coordinator, Janet Mize, the
hepatologist, Dr. Natalie Murray, the chief surgeon,
Dr. Thomas Broughan, the assistant surgeon, Dr.
Viken Douzdjian, and many associates whom I would
meet in the course of testing.

I felt as though I were back in school,
preparing for orals, and praying that I passed in
order to be a lowly candidate, "on the list" for organ

transplantation. This time what was at stake was not some advanced degree, but my life.

In rapid succession, and well coordinated by Janet, I met first with Dr. Douzdjian. I talked and cried. He was young enough to have been my son. This was not the too intelligent to have a liver disease, any disease for that matter, professional self that I wanted to present. I met with a financial advisor. That is when I should have cried. I met with a social worker. I cried again. She, too, was young, but she asked hard questions. I met with the one who would be responsible for my medical treatment, my doctor, in other words, before and after surgery. It was her task to keep me alive until an organ became available. I did not cry, because she told me to call her Natalie, understood my admitted fear and ignorance of physicians and all things medical, including the fact that I couldn't remember my last pap smear, and I wasn't taking hormones because that would have necessitated a visit to a doctor, and anyway she was from my home town, Fort Worth, Texas. I am privileged at this time in my life to call her friend. She was one in my need, and I was impressed by her compassion, her competence, and her brilliance. I would experience the latter on many occasions when, ordinarily conservative in her methods, she would haul out

21

I'm Glad You're Not Dead

(being from Ft. Worth, the predicate applies) some drug intended for an entirely different malady, which was entirely effective, as she knew it would be, but proclaim to me that she hadn't a clue as to why it was working, in order to spare me the clinical jargon. Only she had the credibility to get away with such ambiguity.

When I met Dr. Natalie Murray, I weighed about thirty pounds less than what had been "normal" for me for quite a while, not owing to the blessed, temporary absence of fluid, that too, but from the killing absence of protein in my diet. My head was skeletal; my temples sunken. She immediately prescribed 60 grams of protein a day. I wondered how I could consume that much since I had been scaled down to twenty. An archaic method of treating liver disease is to deprive the poor, dying organ of protein. I can only compare this to prescribing leeches for anemia patients.

At this stage Dr. Broughan, the surgeon, was known to me only by his back, and brisk walk away from my location. He would soon become more familiar. His other predecessors in my candidacy interviews consisted in an ethicist readying me for living wills and powers of attorney. His job was easy. I had already seen to the legal stuff, just in case. A psychiatrist and counselor and I had a nice three way chat. I'm not sure to this day of the precise purpose. I presumed it was to ascertain my relative stability, my potential for endurance, and my attitude for cure. I "handled" the psychiatrist by looking him straight in the eye at all times. I don't know exactly what I expected from this course of action. The poor man probably thought that in addition to cirrhosis, I had a thyroid problem which rendered me bug-eyed.

While I was meeting people, I was concurrently undergoing meticulous and rigorous tests which Janet Mize scheduled with deadly regularity. They took days- utilizing modern state of the art equipment which a university hospital, state supported, can almost afford.

If the narrative has seemed cryptic until now, it adopts a new non-clarity with an outline of what one Janet Mize, R.N., has entitled "Pre-Transplant Evaluation Protocol"--in other words the successive tests consisting in: chest x-rays, ultrasound of the portal and hepatic veins, CT scan of the abdomen/pelvis; electrocardiogram; echocardiogram; labs: CBC, Health Panel; GTT; PT/PTT; Alpha Fetoprotein; Iron Studies; ANA; AMA; Blood Bank Evaluation; Cardiology; angiograms; Hepatitis Antibodies--all of these aimed at a profile of my physical condition and my potential for transplant.

I'm Glad You're Not Dead

This team would not risk an organ, scarce as they are, by housing one in a terminal body. A patient going in must be free from an extrahepatic malignancy, a terminal disease, or an addiction which poses risk from recidivism. Persons with hepatitis, by far the dominant group with liver disease, will retain the hepatitis factor in their systems, and hence carry through life a potential threat to an attack from this source on the new organ. They are, nevertheless, at many centers eligible for liver transplantation--often their only hope for survival. Because for them a liver graft is a treatment, not a cure, many transplant hospitals will no longer accept chronic Hepatitus B sufferers as candidates. Hepatitis B comes back with a vengeance, and the post-transplant treatment is overwhelmingly expensive, necessitating a globulin shot once a week for possibly years. The same is not true for Hepatitis C, which may have persisted in the patient's system for decades before detection, and which does reoccur but has a much slower course.

Testing meant mostly waiting -- sometimes with cause, sometimes not. It was summer and I had much rather been on the beach, well, anywhere really. I felt like Jonah in the belly of the whale, as I was being compelled, much against my inclination, from one port to another. In the beginning I had a

clinician escort. When it surfaced that I lived in
Galveston, I lost that privilege. According to
hospital logic, a weird logo system indeed, because I
was a local, I should naturally know all the twists
and turns of the hospital labyrinth. The fact that I
was a stranger to this complex had no bearing on my
status. I retraced steps often in order to reach the
right elevator, not to mention the correct corridor.
Fortunately, my heart was in excellent condition.

Not only was my heart sound, but so were my
kidneys, pancreas, lungs and other human eco
systems. My spleen was enlarged; my liver
shrunken. I tested out as a viable transplant
candidate. The phone call from Janet, in late summer
of 1993, confirming my acceptance into the program
came as a monumental relief. Dr. Douzdjian said,
upon the initial interview, that if I were accepted, I
would become theirs. I was beginning to realize
what this possession would mean. Once in terror of
transplant surgery, I now felt like celebrating the
possibility. On a low sodium, alcohol free diet, and
with diminished energy, celebrating was becoming
not an event, but a challenge.

I was to discover that I was fortunate in many
ways in comparison with other transplant
candidates. Physically and financially I was better
off than most. I had disability insurance through my

25

university. SSI complemented my benefit to a total of 60% of my former salary. It was, nevertheless, a constant irritant and anxiety to meet my obligations on far less income than I had enjoyed. At the time I was accepted as a transplant candidate I was still teaching and functioning as chair of an academic department. About two months after my evaluation, I ceased working; my energy level was too low, and I was once again experiencing severe fluid buildup adjacent to my lungs. Dr. Murray decided on hospitalization in order to treat the condition more radically than an outpatient status afforded. I left my office knowing that I probably would not return for some time.

Physically, I had not yet experienced periods of encephalopathy, nor extensive weakness. I was still enjoying a relatively normal life, with some days better than others. I was to learn of patient candidates in successive months, whose failing organ function and frequent infections precluded or postponed transplant. I knew two who waited too long to seek treatment and died as a consequence of their debilitating conditions. One underwent transplant after having suffered through postponement of treatment due to religious and ethnic considerations. Japanese and Shinto, his father threatened to disown him should he undergo transplant. The other never made it to surgery. A sweet, dear man, sort of a younger brother to the whole group of liverees, he was initially the victim of a doctor's ignorance or caprice. He experienced pain in the early stages of his disease; his doctor prescribed Tylenol. At this point in the narrative, these two appear as synecdoche, representatives of other cases.

For myself, I began a very long wait for an organ. What I had anticipated to be a period of waiting of about three months stretched into a year and three months.

Chapter Three
What the Liver Said:
Function and Dysfunction

The liver has been called the body's pharmacy; it is also something of a soda fountain. It produces protein and quick energy, stores vitamins, aids in digesting fats, removes toxic substances, regulates clotting and fights infection. It is, to say the least, a complex and valuable organ with some 500 functions in all. It is the subject of people abuse, alone, unprotected, without advocacy or tribunal. 26,000 Americans die each year from liver diseases, the eighth leading disease-related cause of death. Far more than not die of disease in no way of their own making, but the result of others' handling of toxic substances--polluted water, chemicals, needles, blood supplies. Some are the victims of autoimmune disorders. Some are the victims of alcohol or drug abuse, venereal disease, or unknown viruses. 10%

of alcoholics develop liver disease. Cirrhosis, a common condition among liver patients, is the presence of nodules of scared tissue that obstruct circulation of the blood. That obstruction can cause pressure in other organs, resulting in bleeding varices in the esophagus and stomach, and spleen enlargement. Excessive amounts of unprocessed chemicals, toxic to the brain, cause encephalopathy (mental confusion), the extreme form of which is coma. Viral hepatitis also causes cirrhosis.

Obviously, a person with a serious liver disease, regardless of the cause, should not delay treatment and should avoid any and all toxic substances. While six people die every day in the U.S. waiting for a liver transplant, many more die from an acute attack in the case of liver failure. Something as innocent as bacteria in food, raw fish, for example, can result in a fatal infection in the person whose immune system is compromised with liver disease. Death can come very quickly. I know of two young men, both about forty, whose last agonies took only a matter of hours. One, propelled toward death's door by a toxin unknown to me, lived 30 hours. The other, whose death was equally precipitate, ingested raw oysters as a last supper.

What the Liver Said

One should not underestimate the walking time bomb that is a damaged liver. It can literally go off at the slightest provocation.

Bleeds are a chronic threat. The cirrhotic liver cannot supply the coagulating factors necessary to prevent hemorrhaging. I was to experience three more bleeds during my waiting period with about a six month interval in between each. On each of these occasions, I would be driven by dear Ann, on call at all times, to the emergency room at UTMB just a few blocks away from my home where its emergency room crew would attend to me and receive orders from my own doctors. I learned later, nevertheless, that at least once, the team was really worried. Every severe bleed is a serious set back for the patient, and hardly a welcome occurence when one is waiting, indefinitely, for an organ. The emergency room experience is less than pleasant. While many other traumas have already faded from memory, this one is indelibly imprinted. With blood pressure plumeting, my gut heaving lumps of blood, shock setting in, the staff worked quickly and sometimes brutally, at least it seems so on the receiving end. Since I was conscious on all three occasions, I was always naively self-deceptive. Of course, they would save me--they had before.

I'm Glad You're Not Dead

They, on the other hand, knew that I was already in death's arms. I always fought the nasogastric tube, an involuntary response. Anytime the procedure was necessary, I relied on nose lubricants, anesthetic spray and lots of will power. Without the nose tube, draining the blood that collected in my stomach, however, I might have drowned in my own blood.

My veins are naturally small and in medical "poke" terms, they roll and blow, interesting language in another context, not so in ER. While they desperately tried to introduce plasma and other counteractive agents by IV, they discarded needle after needle and abandoned site after site. In other words, I was a pin cushion, with many not so tiny orifices, within a few minutes of anxious treatment. Summary - Ouch! Once under control I was shipped to ICU where I could be closely monitored.

It was after one of these episodes that I experienced a terrifying, yet funny, period of encephalopathy. On the mend, in my own room, while waiting for enough improvement to merit discharge, my routine blood tests indicated a systemic infection--my white cell count, usually below normal, was way up. The cause was unknown; antibiotics were introduced. Somewhere in all the

32

What the Liver Said

treatment and orders, whether because of the shock and weakness pursuant to the bleed, or counteractive medication, I lost it. The encephalopathy was extreme for at least 24 hours, and never quite absent again.

In the course of one night I was a little nuts. Ann had been to see me in the evening, and had left for the night. I was aware after a few hours of la la land that she was gone. I panicked, not remembering that she had gone home and had told me so. I was worried about her since she was a smoker, and the only place to smoke on the hospital grounds was a shadowy bus stop, poorly lit, and some distance from the madding crowd. In my confusion, I asked the nurse of her whereabouts and was told that she had left the hospital about ten p.m. In my desperation, I wanted to call Ann at home, to be sure that she was indeed there, but could not remember the number. In no way could I put together the sequence of numbers which I called so often. That lapse was cause for further alarm. I asked the nurse to look up the telephone number and then I had to write it down (not too legibly) in order to retain it. I succeeded, of course, in waking Ann, only to share my alarm at her absence and to ascertain that she had gone home, In the interim that it took her to fall back asleep, I was now on another kick. It had been my habit to call her early in the morning, since hospital nights aren't really nights, and mornings may begin with weighing as early as four a.m. Ann is not a morning person, and any alarm, ringing or cosmic seizure is necessary in order to awaken her. This night I called her back about 2 a.m. to tell her not to oversleep. She is still my friend.

In the course of that same night, and in my confusion, I was aware of being very uncomfortable, all tangled up in sheets and blankets and the infamous hospital gown. I seized upon the gown as the source of all the misery and so tried to take it off. This normally simple feat was complicated by the fact that the IV tube was hampering my getting out of the sleeves. I determined, after great deliberation, that I could slip the sleeve, still a part of the gown, but both now separate from my body, over the IV monitor and pole down to the floor, whereupon lifting the pole slightly, the gown would be free and I could place it under the covers until modesty and some vital signs technician caused its replacement. My tactics failed. I stood awkwardly between the bed and the pole stark naked and shamefacedly rang for the nurse for help. There was, of course, reference to my disturbed state of mind the next day.

What the Liver Said

In the course of the same period of
encephalopathy, I asked for ice, and stipulated that
it not be too cold! Dr. Murray sent the attending
fellow in in the middle of that bizarre night because
she thought that the central line, still in my neck,
from ICU, might be the source of an infection and
the cause of the symptomatic psychosis. He removed
the line, and several layers of skin with all the tapes.
In bandaging the site, he asked for a 4x4. With my
sense of humor still intact, and not entirely in
confusion, I asked what on earth was he going to do
to me next, as I envisioned a 4x4 board, and
someone swinging it at my head. I guess I felt that
somehow the act was appropriate. There is a lot of
black humor among liver patients over seiges of
encephalothopy. It is treated with varying doses of
lactulose, a drug which, while softening the stool and
acting as a laxative, also helps eliminate "bad
humors" from the bloodstream. "Pass the lactulose,"
is frequently echoed in clinic and support meetings.
It is the "in" joke.

Some get stuck in prolonged states of
encephalopathy awaiting transplant. A symptom of
this state, perhaps the main one, is forgetfulness.
The behavior pattern is not unlike the early stages
of Alzheimer's disease. Patients have related

35

incidents of not knowing where they were or how
they got there, or more frightening, how to get
home. Some confuse articles of clothing. I would, on
occasion, walk into a room, and not remember why I
had gone there. Twice, I had the terrifying
experience of thinking clearly but not being able to
translate the thoughts into speech. Often toward the
end of my long wait, I could not lay my tongue to the
right word--I would hesitate, and often another
supplied the word for me. This particular symptom
of my disease was a source of great anxiety and
frustration for me. I had always been quick,
articulate, with a well developed and exercised
vocabulary, perhaps the most articulate of anyone
in my circle. Now I was sputtering. My anxiety
extended to the future. I earned my living by
manipulation of language. I was a teacher of
literature. I loved words and loved to use them.
Now I appeared to myself to be some kind of
borderline idiot. Self-esteem dissolves with this
illness. Proportionately a support system, beginning
with self, is preeminent.

One must keep reminding one's self that all this
will pass -- that after transplantation, health and
faculties will be restored. If ever positive thinking is
applicable, it is at this time, the time when one feels
weakest and a little, or a lot, lost. Discouragement,

What the Liver Said

sometimes depression, must be fought as far greater enemies than the disease itself. I am a little shy at revealing my own psychosomatic practice during this interminable seeming waiting period. I went through the predictable emotional highs and lows, more lows now, I recognize in retrospect, than I addressed at the time. Each patient has his or her own coping mechanisms. Mine seemed to me then and now as more than a little presumptuous.

Still, my life was entirely on hold, and entirely out of my control, a facet of this whole ordeal which was probably the most odious to me. Not only did I meekly have to follow doctors' orders, but I had to clear ordinary aspects of my life, activities which I had always presumed and enjoyed at will -- such as driving, spending time in Houston, or visiting my family in north Texas with my medical oligarchy. I really had to undergo a personality transformation; independence and autonomy had characterized me formerly. I was, to wit, a proud, stubborn Leo, reduced to a dependent state. And, to tell the truth, I felt some trepidation and weakness on my own, second thinking activities which I would have barrelled into naturally. I worried about walking on the beach bare-footed for fear of infection, and yes, in spite of my rebel protestations, I did worry about driving.

I'm Glad You're Not Dead

Dr. Murray, toward the end of the progression of the disease, told me very forcefully not to drive. She worried, quite justifiably, about an episode of encephalopathy in which I might not realize that I was running a light, or driving on the sidewalk, or God forbid, over someone. This was the only proscription of hers which I disobeyed. Like so many people whose independence is identified with driving, I could not give it up -- to do so would seem like giving in, perhaps, perversely, even giving up. But I was anxious.

So for several months, I lived alien to my former, gregarious, self-confident self. I had always rejoiced in good conversation with close friends, and was blessed to have a circle of warm, witty, intelligent ones. Now I sat in their midst, self-consciously, paranoid even, that my slow translation of thoughts into words, or my eclectic management of them would be noted. Reluctantly with a group I turned the steering wheel over to another "designated driver," and alone I worried about the future. My dark nights of spirit consisted of complaining aloud, usually to faithful Ann, that I would never, after transplant, be normal again. I envisioned some form of semi-invalid state, unable to work, physically weak, devoid of playful outlets,

What the Liver Said

exercise, travel, afraid to be far from medical care. I
voiced the concerns in an effort to exorcise them, I
think. I hoped that if I spoke them, I reduced their
probability. I recited my future pitiful limitations
like a canon each time that I was down. I was
charming company.

On the other hand, mercifully, and more
constantly and solidly than the negative periods,
was a platform of hope and faith. I was, in some
private and very firm foundation of my being, sure
that everything would be all right. I told myself
that I would ace it -- that surgery and recuperation
would go swimmingly, that I would recover faster
and better than anyone else had. This optimism was
not the offspring of pride, but of self-determination.
I did pray, and I did rely on the benignity of a
generous Father. I had never thought of God as
some kind of cannibal, and was certainly not going to
start now. My chief tenets of religion consisted in
His unconditional love and my willingness to do or be
whatever it was that I was to do or be after surgery.
I believed that I would be O.K. I never harbored the
notion of dying; I did not accede to the possibility
even momentarily. I dismissed it. I practiced for
the first time in my life a degree of formal mind-
control. Some of my good friends, more given to
psychic mind games than I, loaned me tapes on self-

hypnosis. I did utilize them enough to learn to relax on cue, and block out distractions or destructive, even painful, stimuli. I would recommend similar exercises for anyone awaiting transplant. One efficacious result is the feeling of being in control again, at least to a degree, of one's life. If I could not control the what, when and how much of medication, the frequency of clinic visits, the occurrence of symptomatic trauma, the occasional nausea, or weakness, the excessive urinating, diuretic-induced, in short, the fraility of my body, I could control my mind, and therefore my attitude, and to a significant degree, my emotions. So for morale's sake, I could counterpose having to postpone any activities beyond running distance of a toilet until after the morning's diuretics had run their course, against my attitude that all this was an adventure, especially the anticipated surgery, and its mysterious aftermath, one which I had never experienced and which I looked forward to as a new phenomenon, one from which I could grow and learn. It is true that what lurked in future shadows was indeed a mystery for me. Until this illness I had never been hospitalized, and so it goes without saying, I had never had surgery. There is at least irony in circumstances that presented me with my first operation room experience in the form of

What the Liver Said

surgery that was to last ten hours, include every
life support available, and use more than 60 units of
blood.

I waited fifteen months for an organ match. In
order to transplant a donor's liver, the new organ
had to "match" the recipient in size and blood type.
In liver transplant a tissue match is not required.
One of my last memories in the OR before I was "out,"
was a sincere, eager young resident who, in an effort
to cheer me up, leaned over and whispered that this
was a good liver and a good tissue and blood match. I
do not remember if I only thought, or said aloud,
that one of us was in the wrong OR and I fervently
hoped that it was he, since there is no tissue match
in liver transplantation.

In part my long wait was due to my blood type,
in part my size (I am not a "large" woman - my chest
measurement determined this aspect) but mostly, as
with all cases, the long wait was owing to the
sparcity of donors.

At this point, about five months after
transplantation, my writing was interrupted for
more than a month because of another illness, not
mine this time, but Ann's mother's. In a weak
attempt at offering my friend some assistance in a

concern of hers, after her surpassing loyalty to me, I accompanied her and her mother to the Cleveland Clinic for diagnostic purposes. The trip took us first to Kentucky where Pauline lived, then to Ohio, back to Texas and round trip back to Kentucky, and home again. I recount this journey because it took place about five months after my surgery, and because I withstood the usual fatigues and relative hardships of a car trip, doing at least half the driving, with as much ease or disease as my companions. I had no concern over being so far from my medics, nor over road side food or lodging. With one exception, having nothing to do with my transplant, I fared well. I felt free, useful and "normal." The exception to my well-being consisted of a fall I took in a motel lobby. My dog, in an anxious and intense effort at being the first to exit through the outside door, ran between my legs and tripped me up. I fell hard, on my left side. This animal harbors extreme anxieties about being left behind. Yes, he is the same dog who accompanied Ann to Houston during my comatose period, for which he is not responsible. He is appropriately named Rerun, having been recycled two or three times at the SPCA before he decided on Ann and me as appropriate caretakers. He came cheaply and has since cost us about three thousand dollars. He has an inoperable cataract and a

What the Liver Said

detached retina. He has rivaled me in health care benefits.

I fell with my elbow burrowed into my ribs and emerged with painful brusing in my rib cage. For a month I could not sleep on my left side and most movements were difficult and very sore. I was more embarassed than anything at the time and ascertained on my own, naturally, that there was no serious damage. Back home, Janet suggested with more than just sincerity that I might wear a medical alert medallion. I am considering the possibility. What is interesting to me here is that, whether foolish or not, in the crisis I entered into my old mode of shrugging off an injury, in spite of my immediate medical history. I take comfort in that attitude, familiar and natural as it is, if my doctors do not.

My medical friends and I laughed at the fact that my first real opportunity at venturing out for any significant distance and time consisted in a visit to, of all places, another clinic. Natalie remarked that some people really know how to take a vacation. It was all sweet to me. I encountered spring on this journey, in all its verdance and mystery.

By the time of the return trip, the second time around, Easter Monday, 1995, the dogwoods were in bloom in the Tennessee valleys of the Great Smokies.

I'm Glad You're Not Dead

We drove through the area when the mountains
were hidden in their own "smoke" for it was raining
and the fog was thick. The white blooms were
effulgent and proud in their own distinction,
unchallenged and undiminished by shadows greater
than they. I had taught analogy and symbolism all
my academic life; never had I experienced it so
personally and poignantly. Everything around me,
in this Tennessee mountain home, said resurrection
and new birth -- I was aware of layers of response
in myself, many unexercised and latent, shy, secret,
laboring to the surface of consciousness, dependent
on my effort for their fruition. I was struck by how
far I still had to go to respond appropriately and
proportionately to gifts of life. The same was true in
other areas of my life. I wanted to give more, love
more, do more, amend more, in gratitude and
justice. I was deeply aware that I was just too puny
to act fittingly. The great mountains did not
diminish the gentle, white dogwood flowers, and
they did not, as gift, diminish or reject me; they
lifted me up, while they humbled me out.

The long months of waiting had taken their toll
on my sensibilities. I had, for survival's sake, closed
off many tendernesses, and shut down emotionally.
The wait had been hard, very hard.

What the Liver Said

At about this same time I received a phone call from a support group member, Pete, who had just undergone his first false alarm. Since I had experienced four similar calls before transplant, he wanted me to tell him how I had coped and what he could, now, expect. By false alarm I mean a page or a phone call from Janet alerting the candidate that the long winter of wait might be over. I usually got: "Elizabeth, where have you been?!" on my answering machine, though not the morning it was all for real. Pete had flown in from Corpus, and like me on more than one occasion, had been prepped for surgery, only to be told that the liver was unfit and was, consequently, rejected by Dr. Broughan for transplant. Pete was left looking for a kindred spirit and I was chosen. I was more than happy to do some propping up. Anyone in this sincerely active support group would have been. I shared with him the ambivalent emotions which I had felt after the successive disappointments. He was, as yet, only feeling, not articulating. This experience of a last minute change of plans is not common, but happens often enough that it is covered in a candidate's protocol preparation.

I had reacted with relief on the one hand that I would't have to face surgery with its severe

45

implications just yet, and disappointment that this altogether new side of my adventure was not yet upon me. I also shared with Pete, from my post-transplant vantage, just how fortunate I thought we were to be the beneficiaries of our surgeon's caution and conservatism. I knew that he had his institution's pressure upon him to produce. Dr. Broughan did not take risks with his patients.

As for Pete's second concern about what his false summons might portend for the future, I could neither reassure nor condole. He was simply back on the waiting list, in the pool. Only someone else's demise, someone with a healthy liver at the time of death, with his blood type, and, as long as he remained non-critical, within his region, could change his status permanently. In other words, someone had to die to quiet Pete's own fears about his hazardous state, and that someone had to have signified his intentions to be an organ donor. This critical and crucial trade off of life for life causes not a few organ recipients anguish and unjustified guilt. It also causes immense swells of gratitude.

The procedural aspect of who gets an available organ and when, according to liver coordinator, Janet Mize, R.N., the Super Janet, referred to so often in this narrative, is simple and relatively well regulated. With regard to transplantation, the

What the Liver Said

United States is governed by a non profit, federally
funded, private organization, the United Network for
Organ Sharing (UNOS), which accounts for organs
and their distribution throughout the country. This
"mother company" maintains a data base which is
monitored by the various regions through the U.S.
responsible for this geographic patient population.
In Pete's case, as in mine, our Organ Procurement
Organization (OPO) has access to UNOS' data base, as
do the transplant centers and participating
hospitals. When an organ is donated within a region,
the transplant surgeon is notified. He or she must
be notified if a donation has been made, even though
the medical condition of the donor, or of the organ
may cause the surgeon to reject it on the basis of
the telephone information alone, e.g., the donor
suffered from hepatitis, or was on life support for so
long that the organ function had started to wane.
The transplant surgeon determines whether he and
his team will go into action, whether one of the
recipient's surgeons, or a transplant surgeon at the
donor's hospital, will harvest the organ. Meanwhile,
the listed candidate with the donor's blood type and
with, in the case of two or more of that type, the one
with the greatest need, is called, given whatever
information is available at the time, and told either
to wait for later orders, or if the recipient lives at

I'm Glad You're Not Dead

some distance from the hospital, to begin the journey in, as if he had not already begun it, a lifetime ago.

Chapter Four
"Who Only Stand and Wait. . ."

Upon becoming part of the liver recipient internet, becoming "theirs," as it was put to me initially, I anticipated a wait of from three to six months.

When I left my academic duties in September of 1993, knowing that I was entering the hospital for treatment, and having it suggested that I might remain there long enough for an organ to become available, I made all the necessary arrangements. I lined up my teaching replacements, left notes for my Dean and a senior colleague in my department, and temporarily purloined my office PC. It was possible that I might return in a few days or, as it happened, not for almost two years. Those immediately concerned knew that I carried a pager and was on alert for that terribly important beep. A component of the long wait was the all too frequent false beeps, brought on by wind and rain storms, and random "wrong numbers." The beep initiated panic and action in the early days, and eventually elicited apathy and skepticism. I knew that Janet would call my home first, before using the pager, and since I had an answering machine, and was never out of pocket for long, I adopted a more relaxed attitude, and in fact, much to everyone's chagrin, often forgot the pager itself.

In retrospect I wonder that I was not anxious during a fifteen month listed wait about not receiving an organ in time. I had supreme confidence in my team. I believed that, as they monitored me, increasing or decreasing medications, they would keep me in shape. I complied by exercise, chiefly through brisk walking and some swimming, and my own monitoring of nutritional habits.

As a hobby I watched cooking shows on TV, always with an eye and a pen out, for low sodium and low fat recipies. I compiled copious notes, threw in some of my own ingredients, modified some of the gourmets', and ended up with a compendium of dishes good for what ailed me (and by extension anyone with a liver disease). Ann organized my transcribed mess. Out of it all we probably have a

publishable cookbook. We might, however, have a
problem with documentation and lawsuits. I can't
remember the source of any, and I have modified all
of the dishes. So much for wealth and fame. At any
rate, I hasten to assure all interested persons that
sins of the palate are still possible both before and
after transplant. Life is not just one big sacrifice. I
was, however, naive in my complacency and my
assumptions about being transplanted before it was
too late.

The first time I was put through the drill, I was
beeped on my pager and I was wearing it. I
responded, a little excitedly; dug out Janet's card
with her number on it and returned the page from
the supermarket pay phone where I had been
reached. Something was altogether wrong with the
communications system, so I went through check
out, calmly dissembling, loaded groceries, all the
while thinking this is/isn't for real, and I'd know as
soon as I reached home. Sure enough, the first
"Where have you been?!" greeted me over the
machine. I cannot remember if I was to come in
immediately or wait for further instructions.

I do remember the scenario of the absurd
which took place at home in the meanwhile. Ann and
I kept bumping into each other as we prepared for

51

my indefinite absence from home. I saw to trivial things; all of the important ones had already been seen to. Indeed, we were overprepared. Everything of a legal or financial matter was in order. Since I had just been food shopping, there was plenty in the house to eat--alas. I had purchased, as usual, my succulent fresh fruit, which I would be forbidden to eat for some months after surgery. Because of potential for infection from sources such as fecal matter in water, pesticides, etc., liver transplant patients must abstain from uncooked fresh fruit and vegetables for several months after surgery and from sneeze bars forever, and follow a regime of washing fresh fruit and vegetables scrupulously. On the occasion of the summons, as on succeeding ones, I had to go NPO, i.e., nothing by mouth, food or liquid, even water, until after surgery, sometimes a matter of days after the initial call.

This first time was exciting and a little, not a lot, scary. Not having been through the drill before, I presumed this was it, and I wouldn't be home again for quite a while. I effectively told my home good-bye, well mostly my ocean view, and walked bravely out the door. I mean I walked bravely out the door; it was a considered pose. Now that I think of it, I compare it to only one other such moment in my life -- when I knelt in my parents' kitchen to

52

"Who Only Stand and Wait. . ."

hug my eleven month old brother, David, before
adopting another considered pose, and walked out
the back door to join the convent. I have long since
abandoned that vocation, but apparently not my
predelection for walking self possessively out of
doors.

Ann drove me to the hospital, only a few blocks
away; this time to its front door, not to the
emergency room, where I had stumbled in so often
before, after bleeds, and in a real panic. She
dropped me off and went to park. She, too, was
extraordinarily calm. I, quite familiar with the
place, reported in to the sixth floor, Ward B, to find a
room and a familiar nursing staff waiting for me. We
were old friends. It is an anomaly that I would walk
briskly, energetically through the halls and to a
room where, by that passage, I would immediately
become a patient, even one with only percentages of
surviving the next few hours, being acted upon by a
friendly but efficient team.

Surgical prep is enough of a common
experience for the population that I will not detail it
here. For the liver transplant patient the only
unique procedure is the introduction of an IV for
purposes of hydration. Naturally, and returning to
the strange logic of a hospital, the IV was introduced
before the enemas and shower. That made perfect

sense because then I could run to the toilet, after falling over the pole, or frantically dragging it behind me. Similarly, I could shower holding one bacteria ridden arm outside the stall. Once again, I was nudely connected to an IV pole, this time in possession of my faculties.

All the while Janet, in the midst of coordinating blood supply, OR arrangements and supporting staff, reported in at every stage of the game: Dr. Douzdjian was at the donor hospital waiting for the heart surgeons to complete their task; he ascertained that the organ looked good; he was on the plane on the way back; surgery should begin in about two hours. Natalie (Dr. Murray) poked in and out; she distributed her very welcome presence between being the doctor and playing mother. At one time in our eclectic conversations, she reminisced about her youthful antics with a pack of friends from our hometown of Ft. Worth. It seems she and they had just finished reading Tristen and Isolde in senior class English, and being on Lake Worth on a weekend, had determined to build and sail a Viking burial ship. The reader should know that a Viking burial ship is set sail aflame. Of course, they drew down upon themselves the wrath of various parental and emergency departments, not to mention the Strategic Air Command (Lake Worth adjoined Carswell Air Force Base). We laughed, and then it occurred to me, and I remarked to her, that I really appreciated her talking about burial ships at this particular moment in my life! She could have picked some other topic with which benignly to distract me.

By this time it was the afternoon of the day following Janet's evening phone call. Ann and I were waiting in my room, alternately watching TV and talking. I had been x-rayed and had blood drawn. I had determined that neither my parents nor my sister, Margaret, were to be notified until I was actually in surgery, and only after then, of course, were others close to me, another sister and brother included. My reasoning was that I had been warned that recipients had been prepped before only to be told that they should get dressed and go home; the organ was unacceptable. My parents, well up in years and my father's sight failing, would have to drive some six hours to get to me. I did not want that effort to be for nothing. As it happened, my judgment was confirmed. Back in the lab at UTMB, the transplant surgeon, Dr. Broughan, detected a laceration, not readily seen, in the donor liver. By this time I was on a gurney in the holding room outside the OR. The anesthesiologist had just begun an IV drip "to relax" me and I was alternately snoring and talking with Ann, in her lovely greens, and with others, and staring at the original murals on the ceiling above. Various pediatric patients had painted them. It still strikes me as strange that these fantasy images hovered above patients about to go under. Mermaids, Disney characters and one really threatening monster, combination high tech and high myth floated above me. I was not surprised that post-transplant patients sometimes hallucinate in ICU.

I had not seen Janet since she passed by in the hall, outside the holding room, carrying a large Igloo cooler. Abruptly, in the middle of my peaceful, snory puffs and attempts at brave humor, the team appeared like the three monkeys -- see no, speak no and hear no. I have the greatest respect for this medical team, and I know I appear irreverent, but at this point I was the observer and their humanity was hanging out. They were more disappointed than I, and I venture to say, even a bit apologetic, certainly chagrined, and maybe embarassed at having to tell me it was a no go. The organ was damaged; they couldn't chance it.

I was sent back to 6B to have the IV removed, whereupon I was free to dress and leave the hospital.

"Who Only Stand and Wait. . ."

My immediate reaction was very basic -- I was
thirsty and hungry in that order. I had had nothing
to drink or eat since the evening before; almost
twenty-four hours had elapsed. Though we lived
only a few blocks away, we went directly to a
favorite restaurant and drank about a gallon of iced
tea, ate, went home and fell, exhausted, into real
sleep. My needs were simple and so was my attitude
-- something like Vonnegut's Billy Pilgrim on his
journey: "So it goes.

Chapter Five
"Postcards from the Edge"

I went home to wait. I was into the second summer of my discontent, actually in better shape, thanks to my maintenance program of medication, than a year before, but frustrated and anxious. Given the fact that I had lived my life by semesters for years, the summer always suggested a certain different, though repeated, rhythm - travel, leisure, freedom to pursue reading, hobbies and rest. Well, I had had quite enough of the above to last a lifetime, with the pulsating exception of travel. I was restricted to the beeper's edge, a grand circumference of roughly ninety miles.

I could still enjoy what was closely available to me -- the beach, swimming, crabbing, and occasionally playing tourist by touring an original pre-turn of the century Galveston mansion, tuning into all the stories of the Great Storm. What my

mother had always referred to, directed at my
father, as the Parr itchy feet syndrome was,
however, rapidly taking on centrifugal force. I
determined that, list or no list, (I had made it to the
top simply by staying power -- a kind of seniority), I
was going someplace. Ann was out of school; she
could drive. I had not been to visit my parents and
reassure them about my condition for months,
though they had, as always, generously, visited me.
My condominium apartment, almost surrounded by
water, had supplied me with vistas and changing
scapes. I had frequent supportive and welcome
visitors from among my close friends. I was on the
board of the condominium and so was entangled and
embroiled enough in people petty. Still, I had not
travelled in a year and a half. I wanted to go to Fort
Worth and I wanted, because it was the most
different thing I could do without going too far, to go
across the border into Louisiana to Merv Griffin's
gambling casino. I am fiscally rather conservative
and no gambler really, but I wanted (needed) a head
change.

I imagine that patient rationalization is a
syndrome that doctors fear the most. I was good at
it. They knew that, but I was mostly restrained. I
also still had enough gift of gab to talk people, if they
were disposed, into my way of thinking. This was a

tough bunch to crack, but occasionally I managed - or they let me appear, to win. Janet seemed amenable, Natalie too, surprisingly. I was beginning to make arrangements when I received a call at home. Janet had run this wild hair past Tom Broughan, whereupon he had, in Texas colloquii, had a cow. No one, it seemed, who was at the top of his region's list was going anywhere. Message sent and received. I wasn't going anywhere.

I adjusted pretty well and continued my routine, slightly limited, activities. One summer day Ann and I had to go to Houston on business. That metropolis was only 50 miles away and so I was allowed. The rule of thumb in transplant travel arrangements is that one should, ideally, be no more than five hours away, by whatever mode of transportation, from the transplant center. This temporal constraint is a factor of a contingency of greater moment. A liver is viable only up to about eighteen hours after harvesting. This length of time is fortuitous in that it allows a window of opportunity for a second or even third option for an organ taker. If the first listed recipient's surgeon rejects the offer of an organ for whatever reason, there is time for acceptance by another, possibly for someone critical, for whom a stop gap graft, even with an inferior organ, can be salvific. If there is no taker, the organ may go to a laboratory for research purposes. The institution who initially or finally uses the organ absorbs the cost of harvesting. In no case, ever, does the donor family pay for the surgical harvesting procedure. There is some confusion about these fiscal considerations, because the heroic methods of life support and treatment, whether surgical or medical, introduced at the end, in an effort to save a life are, of course, charged to the patient's bill, and can easily be read, or misconstrued, as a charge for donation.

Well, Houston was only one hour away, so I could undertake this stimulating journey to a smelly system of freeways matched only by L.A. Or maybe Chicago. In a kind of mild tantrum over Dr. Broughan's Daddy-like control, I got it into my head, I think at Ann's evil suggestion, that I should send a post card to the home team from Houston.

I chose one with an especially snarly sky view of the Houston freeway system, certainly no tourist attraction, appended a note to Janet asking her to say hello to Dr. Broughan, and telling the whole bunch that I wished they were here. The humor and the sarcasm grew and so each day for a few days following I sent a postcard from the following places, circumferance about four miles from the hospital, with a salient note, and always , a "remember me to

"Postcards from the Edge"

Dr. Broughan": Galveston's 61st street pier, my
condo loverlooking the beach, the UTMB "Old Red"
building (archaic medical school facility) and the
Galveston-Bolivar   ferry boat.

I even plotted how I might be able to go on the
ship that sailed out of Galveston for day-long
cruises. This notion entailed logistics involving
helicopters, dinghies, cellular phones and the like,
should I be paged. All of this was entirely too
exhausting, so I settled for the "Texas Duck." The
Duck was a transformed amphibious vehicle designed
as a tourist trap, which toured the Galveston sea
wall by wheels, and then majestically entered the
waters of the bay for a very short, very slow trip.
Were I beeped, I could always swim ashore.
Increasingly I was bumping up against my mortal
limitations. It was beginning to seem as if I really
couldn't do much of anything anymore. I hasten,
however, to juxtapose my gratitude for what I could
still do, against my restrictions.

Many of my friends in the support group have
had it much worse. I'll turn to their voices a bit
later in this labyrinthine narrative. I think of
Charles, the first recipient in the new UTMB
program. He recalled bumping into walls and doors
at the machine shop where he worked, the object of
concern on the part of some, and the ridicule of

others, some of whom thought he might be drunk. The pattern and the image does not fit this large, gentle man, who is always the first to extend his story and his help to new candidates. And Bill, who came into the program after too long a delay, so encephalopathic that he could barely sit up. He had to be strapped into a chair, in which he kept falling asleep during his candidacy interview.

And Judy, who is still waiting some three years after diagnosis. First she waited in San Diego as a candidate in a program that went belly up, now at UTMB where she is alternately on and off the list due to the deterioration of her health, which seems to come periodically, like the monthly "curse."

In Thomas Broughan's own words though an interview with me, he said: "How I view the candidate has changed, and I think will always change. I feel a little bit constrained in that because we are so carefully scrutinized in terms of outcome, and in terms of cost, I worry always that what we do as the result of external pressures may not be what we should be doing in terms of practicing the pure art and science of medicine." When I asked him to be more specific, he simply said: "Yes. Patients who don't have money. The whole health care debate has really drawn that into sharp focus. When patients see me, they are going to die if I can't help them,

and if I can't help them because they don't have the
money, that's a terrible feeling."

Most people do not have the money; many do
not have the insurance. There is the case, for
example, of a fifty three year old African-American
man, treated by a hospital which did not even list
him as a candidate, though he believed that he was,
for six wasted months, who, finally, learning of his
status, presented himself to UTMB only to be told
that he would die; that now, certainly nothing could
be done for him.

The United Network for Organ Sharing (UNOS)
is currently revising its methods of distribution.
The result should be more equitable with regard to
persons and locations. In the current system in
which the country is divided into regions, people
who are financially well off can exercise the privilege
of multiple listings just by reason of their access to
transportation. And, as with every human
institution, politics hold sway. Unless carefully
monitored and held accountable, doctors, hospitals
and OPO's could easily slip into a syndrome in this
country whereby the poor people donate the organs
that the rich have access to. As I write this, across
the country, organ donations are scarcer than at
any time in recent history. This fact alone, an
indication perhaps of a cynical attitude on the part

65

of some, means certain death for others. More than 5,000 Americans are standing at the door of death awaiting a liver transplantation. More than 42,000 await a kidney, liver, pancreas, intestine, heart or lung. In 1994 fewer than half of those waiting received an organ. What happened to the other more than 20,000, and why?

Chapter Six
"The Final Summons"

There were to be three more calls from Janet before the big one. In two cases I went through the whole surgical prep routine again. In one, Janet called regularly to keep me informed of stages in the harvesting procedure, but was able to tell me before I had to leave for the hospital, that the liver was fatty, and therefore unacceptable. A fatty liver can be the result of a donor's nutritional habits. In America's society of greasy fast food and abuse of alcohol, some persons have fatty livers; it is not life-threatening, but not donor friendly, either.

Two of these alerts were only about two weeks apart; all of them occurred within a time frame of about three months before the real event. Finally, Sunday morning, October 23, at 6 a.m., Janet's call came just as I was about to take my first sip of coffee. This time she did not have to ask where I had been. I had been in bed. Once again, she said, "We have a liver for you, and it looks really good." I replied, "I've heard that before." Her reply did carry a measure of conviction. Had I not been there so many times before, I would have been genuinely excited by some elusive but convincing element her message. She seemed convinced; I guess. Once again she laid out the routine: do not eat or drink anything. Wait for her next call. This time, eyeing the coffee cup, and thinking of times before when I waited for hours before consuming anything, headachy usually from no caffeine, I reached for the cup. To heck with it. Sure enough, that would be the last cup of coffee I would have for a week. A little disobedience had generally worked for me in life.

Janet called again after Dr. Broughan arrived on the donor scene and had more information about his condition. He was the victim of a gun shot wound, about twenty-six years of age. Fortunately for me, he carried a donor card and had notified his family of his intentions should anything happen to him. Upon being notified of his condition, they had already forwarded their permission, indeed their desire, that doctors proceed with organ procurement. All of this procedure sounds so

"The Final Summons"

clinical. Behind it lives the grief stricken family
mourning the loss of a young son. They would not
have opted for this trade. There are those recipients
who struggle with cause and effect in this situation.
I have not. It is clear to me that I was not the
primary agent inducing this young person's death,
and I live as only a secondary effect. Strangely,
though, while I am prepared intellectually to handle
this as a proposition, I am also emotionally
vulnerable in another dimension. I lost my brother
to a Saturday night special when he was only
twenty-seven. I am in a unique positon to
empathize with this donor family, and it is at this
level, that I respond emotionally. My subsequent
letter of thanks to them, conveyed anonymously, is
the most difficult and most sincere letter which I
have ever written.

The chief surgeon, Dr. Broughan, himself had
flown to Dallas to harvest the liver. Because of this
circumstance, his assessment of the donor's
condition and the organ, from the hospital on the
other end, was as good as conclusive. His evaluation
that the liver looked good was the same as a thumbs
up signal. Things moved fast after Janet received his
tentative word.

I arrived at the hospital about ten a.m. to the
usual flury, by now old hat. This time I had

performed part of the surgical prep at home. I had showered with a disinfectant soap which Janet had recommended, and taken the required enemas. I was determined not to repeat the IV routine. I had only to be x-rayed. The hospital transportation person arrived and wheeled me to radiology, whereupon, after being seen by the technician, I was left waiting in the hall. Fully clothed and feeling no pain, I could not get with the program that left me parked, after the obligatory x-ray, in an area which I knew like the palm of my hand. I judged this to be a silly set of circumstances -- Ann, Margaret and Linda awaited me in my room. I got out of the chair, and pushing it ahead of me, walked back, through several sets of halls and floors to 6B. Once again, nationwide, I had about a seventy-five percent chance of surviving the next twenty-four hours, but I felt fine.

This time I had called Margaret and she and friend Linda had come running. I really believed by now that this was a go. Nevertheless, Ann and I joked about where we would stop and eat on the way home. Natalie was out of town, much to my disappointment, actually with her husband, at a football game of all places. She would be in before the surgery had progressed very far. I missed her bizarre humor and bedside manner, but Janet

"The Final Summons"

compensated more than adequately, and Natalie, as
hepatologist, would be there when I needed my
doctor more than my friend. Janet, meanwhile, was
her usual dynamic self. A ton of dynamite in a
short, sturdy body, she had appeared at the hospital
first in her sailing clothes -- bandana around her
neck, T shirt, shorts and tennis shoes. Everytime
Janet and her husband, David, himself a liver
recipient, try to go sailing, there is a transplant.
Perhaps that fact alone has raised stats at UTMB,
since they are avid sailors. As the afternoon wore
on, she reappeared in scrubs, having just attended
to the thousand behind the scenes arrangements for
which the coordinator is responsible. She kept us
abreast of each event in this complex operation.

The operation is two-fold; I am reminded of a
military theater. Before I was called, the donor
resource team at the other hospital had called the
Southwest Organ Bank, whereupon a nurse trained
in organ assessment had been sent from that
collaborative to assess the donor and get the consent
of next of kin or proxy. The care of the donor was
turned over to that nurse, who then pulled up the
computer list from UNOS' data base. The first on the
list whose weight and blood type matched was the
potential recipient for this donor. His or her
physician was called. In my case, given the

71

"numbers" Dr. Broughan responded positively and flew to the site. The liver of the donor undergoes tests similar to those which the candidate had. The liver must be "healthy." Obviously, the candidate is not.

People move up on the list through attrition, even if they are not critical. Since I had been waiting so long, I had attained this status by seniority. I would have been superceded, however, had someone in my region, with my blood type and approximate size, been hospitalized or next to death at the time. That person would have been classified as a 1 or 2 in the numerical system, and might be in ICU, on a ventilator and experiencing bleeding, at least.

This numeration, 1, 2, 3 and 4, as signifiers of the patient's condition, 1 being the most critical who, in the ordinary course of things, was currently in ICU, and in the bad state described above, is an element of UNOS' attempt to regulate the appropriation of organs.

A four is at home, stable, capable of activities of daily living (ADL), with some signs of liver dysfunction; a three is at home, but manifesting more frequent medical problems; two is in the hospital for at least 5 days with liver related problems. The status one patient is in ICU, not

72

simply to be monitored, or have favorable nursing care, but because he or she is dying and it is for this very sick person, hypothetically, regardless of money, political connections or race, that the call goes out nationwide.

While I remained a three, at home, and capable of activities of daily living, my condition was deteriorating. I seemed better than when I had first presented myself at UTMB, but no one could foresee when I might become unstable, even critical. The doctors worried that every time I experienced a bleed, I took longer to bounce back. Dr. Murray had forestalled the gastric hemorrhaging from portal hypertension for a few months now, with her treatment of octreotide injections. This therapy made me extremely nauseous, and so she kept reducing the dosage until one day she remarked that at some point, I would just pass the vial under my nose and whiff it. This form of ingestion would have been all right with me -- better than the self-inflicted needle wounds I was enjoying - I told Natalie that my thighs looked like I was having rough sex. No such luck.

Both the threshold of pain and the coping mechanism of the liver transplant patient must be very high before and after surgery. Drugs are the dread. All of them have ghastly potential side effects. Before surgery, patients go around nauseated from the lactulose, swollen from the disease, and frequently confused from encephalopathy. The long wait is not some pleasant euphoria from which one will emerge a whole person. One will simply adopt a whole new drug regime with its attendant demands and adjustments after surgery. Still, surgery is the hoped for objective. Now I was about to attain it.

Janet did rehearse what I might expect upon awakening in the ICU after the transplant. She had detailed the tubes and all the other paraphanalia before. I anticipated a room of horrors, something out of a sci-fi B movie. I would be, at least in appearance, the bionic woman. It was this scene that I was trying to spare my parents. Glenda, Bill's wife, had taken a picture of him in all of his post-op splendor. I always wished, after I had seen it, that I had not. That picture alone heightened my anxiety. Janet's words remained relatively abstract; that picture was too concrete. Bill looked like he had metamorphosed into a vacuum cleaner wearing all its accessories.

The anesthesologist did not visit my room this time either. That chat, too, would have been redundant, and I trusted that an M.D., duly certified, would be in charge. A young intern did, along with

about a thousand others, do a pre-op exam. And I
had the obligatory EKG.

I had forgotten, somehow, that fellows and
residents, and maybe even a general surgeon or two
would troop in to get their hand on, or in, as the
case may be. They reminded me of my students and
that identification never recommended them. This
time I had forgotten, at the precise time when young
Dr. Kennedy showed up, red-haired, tall, and looking
like he was fresh from Hyannis Port or some port
around Boston, what Ann and I had concocted at
home. I had, as I mentioned before, a herniated
navel, the result of water retention. I hated it; it
seemed to me obscene, an abnormal distortion.
Probably I projected onto this visible sign all the
disgust I felt for this disease. My spider veins were
apparent; my complexion still a bit jaundiced; my
skin excessively dry, but this "Outie" was my
obsession. I was sure it could be seen through my
clothes. I purchased endless types of waist reducing
athletic garments in an effort to suppress it. It
would not go away. While the doctors worried about
the potential for infection, I exercised castration
fantasies. I had been told, however, that it would be
taken care of in surgery. So, part in jest and very
much in earnest, I had had Ann, after my homestyle
surgical prep, draw a circle with iodine around the

75

navel area and an arrow and inscription which said "fix me." This message was to be, I hoped, the first thing to catch the surgeon's eye in O.R. I had forgotten about this timely inscription when young Dr. Kennedy appeared to punch around on my abdomen. This was our first, but not our last encounter. He kept the composure he had been taught to keep, in the midst of a bunch of guffawing middle aged women, any one of whom could have been his mother. In the OR, however, it was the staff's turn to be raucous, and they were, while I was out like a light. I received the anticipated response. The belly button was repaired and now looks almost normal. Strange that the ugly, pronounced horseshoe scar across my abdomen does not bother me as much as that navel protrusion did. Grist for the analyst's mill.

As I waited now in my room on 6B, adorned in the hospital gown which I had dubbed my Easter dress (I had been hospitalized previously for a bleed on Easter), things seemed to be moving toward a conclusion. Increasingly, I believed that there would be a transplant. My anxiety level did not rise, probably because so far I had not had to undergo any unfamiliar procedures. I was calm, as were Margaret and Ann. We had our M.O. down. Margaret would call Mother and Dad after I was out of surgery to report that I was alive and well and tell them to come on down. At my insistence the poor dears were not to see me until I said -- my reason being that I did not want to scare them in my new form as a vacuum cleaner. So they were to wait until some hoses were pulled.

Perhaps it is time to let the reader in on the joke, which, believe me, is not visually humorous. In most cases, some, or all, the following are in order: an endotracheal tube is placed in the wind pipe and attached to a ventilator; a nasogastric tube in inserted through the nose into the stomach to drain secretions; a catheter is placed in the bladder. Three tubes are placed in the abdomen at surgery to drain blood and fluids from around the liver. Those remain in place for about a week. A T-tube is placed in the bile duct in order to drain the bile into a small pouch outside the body so that it can be measured several times a day. The quantity and the color of bile appears to be an obsession with the staff after surgery. Apparently, it tells them everything they ever wanted to know. The tube is clamped before discharge from the hospital, but may not be removed for as long as three months. Usually, however, it falls out by itself. All of these tubes are inserted after the patient is asleep.

I'm Glad You're Not Dead

Janet was in my room when she received the
call from Dr. Broughan that he was on the plane and
on the way back from Dallas with the harvested
donor liver. I told Janet, teasingly, to give him my
love, and he replied, "Now she says that!" His
response was, of course, in reference to my sarcastic
post cards.

What pops into my mind as I struggle to recall
and relate these few hours is the image of a clock on
the wall outside death row, and that is not what I
felt. I just felt like this is it. I've been preparing;
I'm a little anxious but not much; it will be O.K.
There seemed no need for last tender words, just in
case. I wish that I could make this drama tense,
introduce the element of suspense, recall precise
moments, but it was all like a well rehearsed drill
and I had no doubt of the successful outcome. About
four o'clock I and my IV climbed up on a gurney and
began the roll to surgery. Margaret and Linda
walked with me as far as the elevators; Ann
accompanied me all the way to the holding room
outside the OR. We had waited this long together; we
would wait out the last hour or so with the same
comfortable empathy. I know that it is seemly at
this point to introduce a somber chaplain. No
chaplain. Janet was in and out of the holding room;

the other personnel were unfamiliar. Whatever
communication there was was just passing time.
About five o'clock, in what now seems like a blur,
with little warning, Ann was asked to leave the
room, and I was wheeled quickly through the double
doors into the operating room. Had I wanted to
protest, I had no time. I remember that the room
appeared small and crowded, and then, and only
then, I panicked for one fleeting moment. I turned
to Janet and still, in my execution mode, said, "Well,
this is really it, this time." That profound remark
was followed by the resident's reassuring
information about the tissue match, and I was out.

The surgery lasted ten and one half hours and
I used over sixty units of blood products. Liver
transplant surgeries vary from six to eighteen
hours in length. The disparity is owing usually to
two factors: whether or not a bypass is performed
in order to maintain kidney function and blood flow
from the lower extremities, and with how much ease
or difficulty the old liver is extracted. The old liver's
desperate attempt to cling to its home body is
usually what causes excessive blood loss. Some
livers are more stubborn than others. In my case
bleeding occurred after closing, for whatever
reason, so the surgeon had to go back in, not an
uncommon occurrence. Dr. Broughan did not open

again, however, until after I was conscious and protesting as much as I could given the presence of the endotracheal tube, the anesthesia, restraints, etc., etc. In my mind the thing was over with, and let's please leave it at that, thank you. Janet had warned me before surgery that she was going to leave the endotracheal tube in as long as possible because that way I couldn't talk.

When I awoke very soon after I was in SICU and "cleaned up," I was asked several questions to test my degree of alertness. I can remember them, so I must have been aware and conscious. They all had yes and no answers, so that I could simply nod. I had thought that I would awake with anxiety, wanting to know my exact condition, but I was not anxious, nor even curious. When Ann was finally allowed in, she gave me what information we had agreed on before - how long I had been on the table, what time it was, how "it" had gone, and whether or not they had repaired my deformity. I was satisfied until I heard the talk above me coming from familiar faces and voices that I was bleeding internally and they may have to go back in. I immediately set out to convince them that this simply was not necessary. As I said, it is hard to be very convincing from a restrained and gagged horizontal position, but I tried. Not only that, Natalie was there and had

assumed her stubborn role in my healing. The fact
that we had grown to be friends, in spite of her
careful professional decorum and emotional
distancing was owing to her being an even greater
control freak than I. It takes one to know one and
there had been times in the past when we had
literally stared each other down. Ann, who is quite
the mimic, does a great sketch of the two of us, toe to
toe, hands on hips, bantering back "yes!" and "no." Of
course, ultimately the Dr. Murray won. I did want to
get well.

I don't know what it is with me and this
bleeding thing. It's not like one can just ignore
bleeding and it will eventually go away. In this
instance I got it in my head that if a certain medical
indicator was present, I would not have to have a
second surgery and that there was a nurse in ICU
who knew of this condition. I am sure that I must
have dreamed up this contingency. The nurse I can
still visualize; the symptom I have forgotten. At the
time her testimony became my obsession. The
doctors hovering over me needed to know all this. I
frantically began signaling (restraints in place) for
writing materials. I couldn't get through to them. I
was, I am sure, red in the face; my eyes were
bulging; I alternately frowned and grimaced. I was
on a tear in a desperate effort to communicate to

them that, if only they could corner that nurse, they would learn something that would preclude a second surgery. All would be well. Meanwhile, they hadn't a clue as to what was causing my contortions. Finally, I prevailed; someone read me. They probably sought out Ann in the waiting room and she deciphered my fit. Dr. Broughan went scurrying off for a pen. Once I had pen and paper, I determined that all that was now lacking were my reading glasses and I could make perfect sense. Once I was adequately rigged I began to write my instructions. They resembled the Bam, Boom and Kazam pyrotechnic illustrations from a Batman comic book. I shoved the notebook away in disgust as if it were all their fault. And this after my surgeon had meekly and kindly run around to fetch me a pen. It was all for nothing, anyway. I found out much later that at the time of this particular tantrum, the second surgery was over with, and except for my disposition, I was doing fine.

After I calmed down, I remembered a time when I was equally adamant about getting my way over something and Natalie had swept through the room proclaiming, "I control the vertical and the horizontal!" Too true. I once gave her a T shirt with that inscription on it. She exudes control from her six foot, healthy, busty build. Her curly, jet-black

"The Final Summons"

hair and dancing brown eyes soften the otherwise
overwhelming presence. And I have seen those eyes
grow very soft on occasion.

I was in the Surgical Intensive Care Unit for
five and one half days. My discharge summary
which covers the surgery and ICU internment reads
as follows:

> The patient is a 58-year-old White female
> with end-stage liver disease secondary to
> cryptogenic cirrhosis who was admitted to
> the Transplant Surgery Service on
> 10/23/94 for liver transplantation. The
> patient was taken to the operating room on
> 10/23/94 where an orthotopic liver
> transplant was performed with a large blood
> loss, but no hemodynamic instability
> experienced intraoperatively. The patient
> required infusion of packed red blood cells,
> platelets, fresh frozen plasma and
> cryoprecipitate. The patient was then taken
> to the SICU where her hemodynamic and
> respiratory, as well as other vital functions,
> were closely monitored. The patient received
> renal dose of Dopamine in the perioperative
> period. The postoperative period was
> complicated by hemodynamic instability which

was accompanied by a fall of hemoglobin and hematocrit. The patient's respirator mechanics remain good. The patient was taken back to the operating room on 10/24/94 for re-exploration. An exploratory laparotomy was performed with clot evacuation and control of abdominal wall bleeding. The patient tolerated the procedure well and there was no further evidence of continued blood loss. Following re-exploration, the patient's hemodynamic and respiratory status remained good. Immunosuppression was instituted per post liver transplant protocol.

I was never in any serious pain in ICU, owing mostly to the severance of several abdominal nerves; I was in extreme discomfort owing to water retention. The ascites set in after the second surgery and was so evenly pervasive that it could not be drained though that procedure was attempted. As the tubes were pulled, and I lost my identity as a vacuum cleaner, I turned into the little Pillsbury dough girl. Well, that's what I looked like; I felt like Kafka's cockroach. Like Gregor, I eventually allowed people, including my mother and

"The Final Summons"

father, to be around me. Supportive, as always,
they were near, comfortably housed in an
apartment in my condominium, but not venturing in
to see me until the second day after surgery.
Successively then, friends from Houston came. I and
my hoses sat up the day after surgery; by the third
day, for long periods of time. I did not anticipate a
set back. I knew all the eventualities, but mentally I
clung to my plan. I would just get progressively
better.

Back on the ward I remained uncomfortable
from the fluid retention for two weeks. Early in this
state I gushed from the incision each time I stood,
coughed, farted or pooped. This indelicacy is
indicative of my new demeanor. Since I was
constantly changing or being changed from wet
gowns and bed clothes, receiving suppositories from
male nurses, and generally impatient with these
activities, I had discharged Virtue Modesty and
Virtue Propriety from my ensemble. In other
words, I stripped unabashedly and cursed like a
sailor. I had never expected that my worst pain
after a liver transplant would be from my
hemorrhoids. It's the little things that get you. I
felt so sorry for the nurses; I hated imposing this
changing routine on their already overburdened
work load. I squirted one nurse through my stapled

incision from about five feet away, so thoroughly that she had to change her scrubs. My kidneys worked well. In fact during surgery, as Janet made her scheduled visits to my family and friends, her commentary and reassurance usually, I am told, focused on my healthy volume of urine. So eventually, with nature's course, a little help from Lasix, and the over-active incision holes, the fluid dispelled and my body size returned to normal. It would take several weeks after discharge for my hemorrhoids to reduce to a tolerable level.

While Janet insists and even simple common sense suggests that every liver recipient undergoes some rejection, my discharge summary does not indicate even one episode of the kind, and I do not remember either attending physician ever mentioning a rejection. I did have an infection accompanied by fever and chills. I was thought to be septic, in medical jargon.

One night I awoke shaking uncontrollably. My teeth were rattling; I was soaked from the usual fluid discharge and freezing from the combination of wetness and an electric fan blowing directly on me. The immunosuppression drugs, prednisone and cyclosporine, caused in me something akin to hot flashes, so I kept the room at arctic temperatures. I was not aware of a fever, but I had one of about two

"The Final Summons"

degrees above normal (38.6 degrees Celsius); any infection is to be taken quite seriously when a patient is immune suppressed. The nurses acted swiftly and intelligently.

Dr. Broughan was called; he in turn called back repeatedly; ordering antibiotics and inquiring of my status. I managed to keep him awake all night. Near morning the decision was made to move me back to ICU for closer monitoring. This move seemed to me to be a step backward. I wasn't happy but I wasn't objecting either. I had promised myself that I would be a very good patient so that I would heal and gain strength quickly, and when discharged, would not have to come back in as so many do for "tune-ups." I did not want to go home until there was no doubt that I was ready. So I revisited SICU while cultures grew and IV's dripped and tests were run. I showed Gram positive cocci with coagulase negative staph in the blood and enterococcus in the urine as well as positive stool cultures for clostridium difficile In other words, my bodily fluids weren't just swell on post-op day #11.

I had been biopsied on day #8. There was no sign of rejection. The biopsy was a little scary and the aftermath uncomfortable for one must lie on the right side, immobile, for one hour to prevent bleeding. A biopsy is one of those procedures performed on a liver only when absolutely necessary, because it is a vital organ and because of the fear, especially in a diseased liver, of hemorrhaging. So, while it is a simple procedure in and of itself, it is threatening. Once again I had to sign one of those "I may die" documents, and be reminded of my mortality.

I had never had a liver biopsy. All the information determined about my disease had been the result of blood tests. I would not let the first set of physicians touch me -- some graceful instinct, I guess. If that gastroenterologist were as inept in surgery as he was in treatment, he would have surely killed me. My UTMB physicians apparently never considered the possibility so late in the game. They knew what was not the cause -- hepatitis. I did not even test positive for exposure to it, hence I had to be vaccinated for it during pre-op treatment. I could not be tested for hemochromatosis (abnormal processing by the body resulting in iron overload) until the organ was biopsied after surgery. It tested negative. There are other possibilities-- but the source of the disease was by transplant so far removed in time that no origin could be determined with certainty, hence the term "cryptogenic" -- or hidden origin. I asked Janet in an interview, while working on this personal transplant history, what, precisely, "cryptogenic" meant to the liver transplant medical team. She explained that it meant that after testing for all hepatitis viruses, and they have all come back negative, they've looked at a biopsy and can't tell; there is cirrhosis present, but they can't discern the origin; then they call it "cryptogenic," medical jargon for "we don't know."

My favorite test during this post-op period of hospitalization was the cholangiogram. This procedure determined the integrity of the bile ducts by a kind of x-ray, and occasioned my other opportunistic tantrum. The problem, as I recall it, consisted in the fact that the cholangiogram was performed on an ironing board. Well, its hospital equivalent. I was subjected to it only a week after surgery when I still weighed in at about 2,000 lbs. of fluid, or so it seemed. Technicians, I discovered, do not know how to handle patients. I was still too weak and heavy to move myself from the gurney to the ironing board and the young turks (students) handling me did not really know how. I was left waiting an eternity; the procedure was unbearably long. There was no place on the board for my arms, and in the middle of the ordeal my bowels finally began to act normally. I was flailing around, muttering, cursing, entirely miserable, not crying because I hadn't cried yet and this particular stress

I'm Glad You're Not Dead

did not seem to merit my first tears, just my
exasperation. I insisted that I could not stand this
any longer; they would have to stop. At exactly this
moment Drs. Murray and Broughan materialized.
Their very pressence and their solicitude calmed me.
Probably, in desperation, the young men around me
had summoned them, but maybe not. This was not
the first such occurrence and it was not to be the
last. I cannot explain how they always knew to join
me during an especially uncomfortable process.
They had appeared once before when, during my
febrile period (I had fever) a CT scan was performed
which indicated a subhepatic fluid collection. Using
CT guidance, a doctor from radiology inserted an
abdominal drain. There was real pain that time.
Blessedly, Dr. Murray allowed some morphine. One
distinct drawback to being a liver patient is that
narcotics are dispensed very sparingly. This is not a
disease for someone who suffers from migraines or
any other chronic pain. Even now, almost eight
months after surgery, I am allowed, for whatever
ailment, no more than two regular strength Tylenol
every eight hours, no cold medications to speak of,
and highly restricted antibiotics in the case of
infection. These restrictions will not change soon, if
ever. Dr. Murray explained that they are, in part,
attendant on the supposition that many liver

patients have a history of chemical abuse and may easily shift dependence to a "harmless" drug.

Back to my guardian angels. Because Dr. Murray had been my attending physician during the long hiatus, though Dr. Broughan had intervened during periods of hospitalization, and perhaps because we shared the affinity of the same sex, I felt I knew where Natalie was coming from with regard to her care of me and her other patients. Not so, Tom Broughan. I knew of his significant reputation, and I knew the persona which he presented with care -- sometimes chatty and informal, always clever and articulate, sometimes cooly professional. If he was in a good mood, he enjoined with the bon mot ; it seemed important that he initiate the conversation with a witticism intended to reveal his hold on the real world. My retort always fell flat. In an interview for this book, he seemed open and candid, though selective and thoughtful, about his medical philosophy. In his own words, he expressed his approach to patient care. Referring to his colleague at the Cleveland Clinic, Dr. David Vogt, he said, "Dave and I in the early days kind of put together a philosophy that there was stuff that Mother Nature was going to do to us and to our patients, that we couldn't control, but we should not let that eventuality force us into making bad medical decisions, and if a person died waiting for a liver, we were always saddened, but we felt even worse if a patient had done poorly, because, in retrospect, we felt that we had taken an unnecessary risk. I guess we adhered to the old medical principle: first, do no harm; don't hurt your patient. Some transplant surgeons feel that they can do whatever they want; no risk is too big. . .I worry about me doing something that will hurt them. . .when I have my opportunity to enter in. I want to know that I am doing what is in the best interest of the patient. . .I know what an incredibly long road it is, that the surgery is just the beginning of the whole process for them. I want every individual I can to be provided a fair start. It's just difficult to look back and think -- well, this person died because I made a wrong call here."

Everyday, while I was recuperating I had the pleasure of the company of two exceptional physicians, and one fine nurse coordinator who kept them on a short leash. I looked forward to their visits. My mother called everyday, not always at the most appropriate times, always lovingly and supportively. Ann came by every evening after school. Margaret tooled over from Houston on weekends. As other friends called or visited, and cards poured in, I realized the magnitude of the

spiritual support which I had received. Lots of
prayers and lots of energies had been focused on my
puny self, and I responded, daily, to all this goodness
by progressive healing and gratitude. I knew how
fortunate I was. My initial emotional state was an
abiding peace. That peace has been lasting, though it
has roughened up a bit as I have returned to the
irritations of normal life, and my own volitile
responses. I wish sometimes now that I could
recapture it in all its pristine calm and simplicity.
The religious community to which I had once
belonged has as its motto: "In the simplicity of my
heart, I have joyfully offered all to the Lord." It had
been a long time since I had dwelt in that simplicity.
Post-op, I returned there to visit for awhile.

About two and a half weeks after surgery, a
daring plan surfaced. I had agreed to give a talk on
organ donation at my university, if I was not yet
hospitalized, sometime during the month of
November. My transplant took place on the night of
October 23-24, 1994. Our nurse health coordinator
at the university telephoned me after surgery to
arrange for an alternative to my presence. I offered
up Janet as a great proxy, and Priscilla (Atwood)
suggested a video interview of me in the hospital, to
accompany Janet's presentation. As the time grew
near this celebrated event, Dr. Broughan said

I'm Glad You're Not Dead

something to Janet like "Why not just bundle her up
and take her along?!" When Janet advised me of this
possibility, I jumped at it, but reservedly, because I
hardly dared to hope. I was still on the antibiotic
Vancomycin for my staph infection -- its course was
a full 14 days, and the T-tube had not been capped.
I wanted to be present at the university for a
hundred reasons. My academic community had been
another source of support for me. I had received
messages from countless colleagues, the
administration had been supportive in practical,
fiscal matters, as well as warmly encouraging on the
personal level, and students had responded in
unexpected ways. The university had held a blood
drive for me; many, many people had donated from
diverse populations on the campus.

I wanted to thank these folks in person, and I
wanted them to know that I was well on the road to
recovery -- that fact, I hoped, being their best sign
of an effective appreciation. Besides, I had a
message to deliver concerning organ donation, and
no one, ever, would now be exempt from hearing it.
So on November 17, 1994, I showed up at the
University of St. Thomas, happily esconced at a
podium again. I was welcomed more warmly than I
might ever have hoped. I told the audience of

"The Final Summons"

colleagues and students that I wanted to hug and
kiss each of them, and I meant it, but my perilous
state of immunosuppression prevented such a
display for the present.

Ann had taken off to drive Janet and me to
Houston. I now assumed the role of Janet being an
invited guest to my university and I wanted to
extend the courtesy of providing for her
transportation. Since Janet's home lay between
Houston and UTMB's John Sealy Hospital, where I was
expected, we dropped her off and took the route back
by the seawall so I could take in the Gulf waves and
breezes again. We also ate hot dogs, parked by the
beach. This was, in my grateful, peaceful mind, as
good as it gets. In view of what I had anticipated it
might have been, I would have called this being well.

What I did not know was that this was a test.
Depending on how tired I was/was not on the next
day, how my "numbers" looked, my benign dictators
might discharge me. Sure enough, while I expected I
would probably be released on Monday, I was
discharged on Friday, Novermber 18, or post-
operative day #26 -- about three and a half weeks
after surgery.

Chapter Seven
"Other Voices, Other Rooms"

Every liver transplant patient's course is unique, both before and after surgery. My story is not generic; it is specifically mine. For the person with a liver disease, hoping to find an appropriate identification in this text, I offer, with their good will and consent, the stories of friends of mine in our liver support group.

First, a word about such a group. Increasingly in our society, people seem to gather together over shared trauma, whether psychological, spiritual or physical. Persons with liver disease are no exception, in fact, tradition may have handed us a greater need to bond together than patients with more politically correct diseases. In a different context, Dr. Murray discussed with me the sad fact that liver disease is something of a medical step-child. Until recently it was thought that it was the

97

result of hepatitis or of the abuse of alcohol. On the one hand, nothing could be done about hepatitis, and on the other, in the case of irreversible liver damage due to the abuse of alcohol, one had already sealed one's fate. Over the last few decades, the one hundred or so other causes of liver disease have been recognized, but are only just appearing in mainstream medical education. So there is a potential stigma associated with proclaiming that one has a liver disease. To the uninformed public that might mean either: a) I'm an alcoholic, b) I play with needles, c) I am somehow subject to dirty water or food, or d) my sexual practices are "abnormal." The perception of the liver patient is not unlike that of the AIDS patient -- he or she must have brought the disease upon himself by lifestyle choices, and therefore "deserves" his fate. Couple this burden of perception with all of the anxiety attendant upon a fatal disease, and the need for a support group should be self-evident.

Similar to other such groups, the liver support groups, available out of all transplant centers and most hospitals, which participate in one or more transplant surgeries, can be a source of both consolation and confrontation. The group's main focus is to support the transplant patient before, during, and after surgery, through whatever means

is in order. It is also an educational system,
providing information, ancedotal and clinical. The
meetings may consist in informational topics
relevant to the disease, sometimes with outside
speakers, arranged by the coordinator. Always
there is an informal period in which patients swap
experiences and exchange helpful hints. The
confrontation is not deliberate; it is a by-product.
The liver transplant candidate is confronted here,
most starkly with all the ramifications of his or her
disease, and actually sees and listens to those who
have come through. In this setting all of the facts,
the realities spill out. I remember the first two such
meetings I attended after my candidacy for
transplant was confirmed. In the first, Bill was
about two or three weeks out of surgery and
attended the meeting. He and the others thought his
presence a great victory. I was amazed that he was
there so soon after transplant, but I also took in the
fact that he was wheelchair bound, connected to an
oxygen tank, and because of the complete oxygen
mask, unable to speak clearly or loudly. Bill was
atypical, in that he had had serious lung problems
before the surgery. Janet, as coordinator, was
listing do's and don't's post transplant -- all the
stuff about fresh food products, and pets and plants.
Some patients began swapping post-transplant

hallucination stories, and before the edifying get-together was over, one of the exhibitionists in the group, for the enlightenment of the new people present, raised his T-shirt to display his irregular horseshoe scar. I left this house of horrors in stoney silence. The foregoing is from the perspective of the new recruit. The second meeting was not much better. Ann asked if I really wanted to go back and I said that I did, because, no matter how scary, I wanted to know everything. Eventually, the presentation fell into place,and I came to realize how important the information gathered was, and how necessary and helpful the bonding and the friendships. Now I am one of the veterans, but because of my initial shock therapy, I am careful to appear with a positive case history and lots of hope for the new guys. There is enough terror present in the disease without invoking too much of black humor and graphic episodes.

Some of the real trauma and case histories appear below. Where possible I have simulated the voices of my friends and co-patients. I decided on a synoptic format, over a Q & A form. I am, as the reader should be, most grateful for the candor and confidence of these folks who have come to be very dear to me. In their stories, someone in the

"Other Voices, Other Rooms"

audience, in need, may find the proper alter-ego, and the near match for empathy and hope.

PETE: TRANSPLANTED APRIL 28, 1995

Pete, of the importunate phone call, did get a liver. I caught him as a captive interviewee while he was still hospitalized, but only a few days before discharge. Actually, at the time, he was looking for me. I had assured him that I had had very little real pain from the surgery itself. His experience had been quite the opposite, and he wanted me to know this fact. I think he wanted to know if I had deliberately led him astray in order to relieve his pre-transplant anxieties. I had not. By the time I visited him, he had almost forgiven what he construed to be my deception.

I have mentioned post-op halucinations before in this narrative, attributing them to other persons. It is true that I did not experience any psychotic episode. Those I alluded to in the beginning of this chapter were, in the words of their subjects, often bizarre, macabre, even threatening. Pete's were not. He recalled for me, awakening in ICU, with an awful compulsion to buy a little boy's bicycle. He wanted to tell the nursing staff that he had to go to Walmart, not to worry; he'd be right back. His personal response to this fantasy is that he says all

101

of his kids are getting new bikes for Christmas. These hallucinations, which can stretch into an extended,but not indefinite period of psychosis, may be caused by anesthesia, or drugs. When the new liver is profused at surgery, large doses of prednisone - a drug which is mind-altering - are injected, and, of course, pain-killers, such as morphine may induce temporary psychosis, too. Pete's dream was sweet. In these rehearsals of post-transplant experiences, there is no pattern, but there may be a correlation between the incidents one recalls and the time elapsed since surgery.

Pete talked with me about his knowledge of his donor, a relatively exceptional phenomenon. Pete hails from Corpus Christi. He remembers seeing an ambulance in his own neighborhood the day before he was called by Janet. A young man, the best friend of his wife's co-worker's son, just nineteen years old, had shot himself. Janet called Pete at 5:30 a.m. to tell him that he had an organ match, and to come to Galveston. The few facts which she conveyed about the donor, including the town of origin, matched what Pete had learned of the untimely death of his young neighbor. No one has confirmed anything, but Pete says he knows. And he says that he wished he didn't know. Pete's last words to me before I left his room that day were:

"Other Voices, Other Rooms"

"How do I deserve this: I've been no angel. I'm just a man."

LUCRECIA: TRANSPLANTED SEPTEMBER 9, 1993

Lucrecia and her husband, Claus, are from Guatemala. Claus is a German born emigré. We became acquainted when I was hospitalized for pleural effusions, on the occasion of my leaving work. She was just a few days beyond transplant and was housed in the room opposite mine in a kind of V-shaped four-plex. She seemed to me to be doing well and was anxious to engage me in conversation, to practice her English, which she had taught herself, many years before. She was the victim of Hepatitis B and C. Since C remains in the system so long before becoming unaccountably active, its origin is always elusive. Dr. Murray theorizes that Lucrecia contracted it as the result of visiting nurses vaccinating small children without sterilizing needles, in a house to house dispensation, a practice extended to affluent citizens in some developing countries. She had carried the virus then, as many do, for as long as thirty or more years.

After a short, virulent illness in Guatemala, Lucrecia was literally dying when she arrived, thanks to Claus' international savvy, in the states and at UTMB.

103

I'm Glad You're Not Dead

While I was in the room adjacent to hers on 6B in September, just after her surgery, she experienced the typical infection, stemming from fluid retention, following many transplant surgeries. She was really out of her head. Before the surgeon opened again to drain the fluids, in her feverish state, she had a party. She dreamed she had won the lottery. Claus, who was one of the most attentive husbands whom I have ever known, had gone home to sleep a little. Lucrecia called her mother, her relatives and friends collect in Guatemala to tell them her good news. She invited them all to Galveston where they would be met by a marimba band at the airport, and served a feast of Guatemalan cuisine which she outlined in a precise and enticing menu. Meanwhile, I was overhearing hysterical laughter and high pitched frenzied Spanish. All I could think of was someday that will be me, sans Spanish, and probably with some university administrator standing at my bed.

Dr. Broughn appeared to find himself the recipient of Lucrecia's lottery largesse. She offered him twenty million dollars for his program. His typical, sardonic reply was -- "We don't need your money, Lucrecia; you'll get the same treatment without it." Claus was summoned, and in his European gentleman's mode, brought chocolates with him to soothe his way with his wife's exhausted nursing staff.

Transplant, as with all serious illness, is very hard on a relationship. David Mize, Janet's husband commented that if you do not have a strong one before the illness, you certainly won't sustain one after the whole ordeal. Claus remarked that Lucrecia is not the same person as before the liver transplant; she does not even look the same. Her hair thinned (an unusual reaction) and when it grew back, it was very different, thicker, courser and with a new direction to the wave and curl of it. Her face is fuller (a steroid side-effect), and her disposition has changed. Claus says that before she was sunny and bright; he called her "my angel" and now sometimes, she is, in his words "nasty."

Her hepatitis C has already reoccurred. Claus monitors her while insisting that she do things for herself. He says simply, "I know so very well that she will live 20 years or more, being careful."

CHARLES: TRANSPLANTED MARCH 21, 1993

Charles was the first liver transplant patient in the new UTMB program. He had been listed at Methodist Hospital (Baylor College of Medicine) in Houston when that program terminated, and both

I'm Glad You're Not Dead

Dr. Natalie Murray and Coordinator Janet Mize joined the new liver transplant program at UTMB, with Dr. Thomas Broughan as chief surgeon in 1992. Charles, necessarily, came along. His is another story of bumps and grinds through the hallways of misdiagnosis.

In 1987 Charles took a pre-employment physical. It revealed that he had had hepatitis. No big deal. An internalist discerned some sign of possible cancer growth. A potential big deal. Charles was told to come back in six months for a blood test. There was no sign of cancer, and since that was the Doctor's blind spot, no liver biopsy was performed, and Charles was sent on his merry way. He attributed fatigue and other minor sysmptoms to aging and long, hot hours. Charles worked as a machinist. He was never jaundiced and did not have the symptoms usually associated with hepatitis.

In 1989 he had another physical. The physician who read the results called long distance from New York to Charles at his work site to tell him to get to a doctor immediately and have a liver biopsy. A gastroenterologist discovered an enlarged spleen and a ravaged liver; Charles had Hepatitis C. Charles had had Hepatitis C for more than 30 years. He recalled possible sources for the disease. He had shot himself in the leg in a hunting accident when seventeen years old, and had his appendix removed two years later. Both these medical treatments involved blood transfusions. And, as a machinist, he had job related cuts and injuries throughout his working life. Whatever the origin, the gastroenterologist told him that there was nothing he could do for him.

He was listed immediately at Baylor, Houston, and then after a wait of six months was transplanted at UTMB, Galveston. Charles has had a series of post-transplant problems, including a leaky bile duct which manifested later than in most patients after surgery, bouts of depression, and difficulties with stress and fatigue upon resuming work. Now after retirement, he seems more relaxed, and optimistic. Still he says that if he had it to do over again, and the "it" included the anxiety of the wait, he would not go through it all again. Nellie, his wife, said that she would not be happy with that choice, but would respect Charles' decision because it was he, not she, who would have to endure. I am not sure that, when I see the way she looks at Charles, she is being entirely accurate in her assessment of her attitude. And when I observed the way Charles looked at his grandson at lunch the day we talked, I am not sure that he would opt to pass a second chance, either.

I'm Glad You're Not Dead

BILL: TRANSPLANTED JUNE 9, 1993

Bill, an auto body man, moved with his wife Glenda, from Missouri to Texas eight years ago. Up until that time he had spent most of his adult life doing what he outlined as drinking, working and sleeping. And . . .doing drugs -- uppers. He often worked 16 hours a day. What started out as recreational habits moved into dependency. He drank to be happy or numb. He took pills to keep going. Twenty-five or so years ago he dropped from about 260 pounds to 145 pounds within two years. He made a lot of money back then and spent most of it on speed to keep going. He had back surgery in 1988, involving blood transfusions, and never got over the surgery. He recalls feeling "crappy" all the time. Eight years ago he decided to quit drinking, and asked his wife, Glenda, to get him some help. Bill checked into a rehab center, stayed the obligatory amount of time, underwent the usual tests, and left under the impression that his liver was fine. No physician at the facility told him otherwise. Six weeks later, he experienced his first bleed.

He received medical care thirteen times in the next year. A doctor informed him that he had liver disease, pumped him full of vitamins, put him on Xanex, and told him, in 1992, that he could not be

108

transplanted, and had only a few months to live. Glenda called her own doctor who put them in touch with a transplant program (Baylor University at Methodist Hospital), in Houston, which is now closed. Bill had to be free of any mind altering drug (in his case the prescribed Xanex) for six months before entering candidacy. Meanwhile, the liver disease had caused shunts (holes) in his lungs, which caused difficult, labored breathing. Bill and Glenda waited ten months for a liver and finally received one at UTMB Galveston in June of '93. When I say "Bill and Glenda," I mean just that. This circumstance is the reverse of a pregnancy, unless of course the organ recipient is the wife. I have not addressed, yet, the role of the spouse, or the lover, or other relative in this ordeal. Clearly, their lives are as upended as the recipient's; the generous, candid conversations with my couple friends in the support group allows me the opportunity to write about the significant other's side.

Bill had it rough after transplant. He says that he was calm at the beginning of surgery because he knew that if it was necessary and warranted, Glenda would have "pulled the plug." I am not sure what contingency he was dealing with here, but the thought sustained him. Glenda stayed with Bill, in his room, the entire time he was hospitalized after transplant. She left only to drive fifty miles to work each day, change clothes at their apartment in Galveston, and return to spend the remainder of the twenty-four hours with Bill. She worked as a pastry chef in a supermarket in the little town of Sugarland, south of the Houston area.

She waited on Bill so long in the hospital that the mode of operation became habit. She says that she still orders for him in a restaurant. The caretaker co-dependency can remain a problem if not carefully controlled. In Bill and Glenda's case it had a lot of understandable reinforcement. The first nine months after surgery Bill was in the hospital more often than not. He might be home for nine or ten days and then have to return because of an infection or complication. Now he is stable, able to work a little at a job as grounds keeper at a place which Glenda manages, and they clearly share life as well as an occupation. Bill, in reflecting on his wilder days, says that "Whatever I do, I'll do it with her -- not a buddy; I'd rather do it with her."

They were candid about their sex life, or lack thereof. They have not had sex since 1991. Their exchange on this subject was typical and almost humorous were it not so revealing in its manifestation of a loss.

Bill: "It wouldn't bother me to do without it. I don't know how she feels. Every time I get after her, it's leave me alone."

Glenda: "Every time he went to the gym, he went to the hospital. I was afraid I'd hurt him."

Bill: "It didn't have anything to do with the hospital!"

Glenda: "After awhile you just go through the day, do what you've got to do and that's it. We haven't talked about it here lately a whole lot."

Problems associated with sexual activity and liver transplant emerged often enough in my interviews that I decided to address it head on, with Dr. Murray's help, as I do later in this chapter. Intervening are other conversations, one of which, with David Mize, approaches the subject of sex again.

DAVID: TRANSPLANTED MARCH 26, 1992

David, as Janet Mize's husband, has little or no anonymity wherever he goes these days, and not in this volume either. He, too, was most cooperative in discussing his case and the issue of sexual function.

111

I'm Glad You're Not Dead

David was, by profession, a fireman, and contracted Hepatitis C while a paramedic with the Houston fire department. That occurred back before latex gloves and cautionary practices in handling bleeding patients. An internal medicine physician could not find the source of his diminished energy and other minor symptoms. The symptoms persisted until finally a gastroenterologist at Methodist Hospital identified the Hepatitis C virus and suggested, rather casually and caverlierly, according to David, that a transplant might be in order three or four years down the road. This was, by the way, the same gastroenterologist who had taken such an indifferent interest in my case. By my time, he was, probably for some very good reason, no longer at Baylor-Methodist, but now at an HMO clinic.

David experienced excessive swelling, lack of stamina, memory lapses, incidents of impaired judgments. Meanwhile, he was driving a fire truck - once, right through a closed station door! He had frequent nose bleeds, had to be hospitalized for ascites. The doctor addressed a possible circulation problem. He continued working, as a very sick man, until he had put in his twenty years toward retirement -- about one and a half years after the occurrence of his first symptoms.

"Other Voices, Other Rooms"

David was transplanted at Methodist before
that program closed and UTMB Galveston's opened.
His surgeon was a student of heart transplant
pioneer, Michael DeBakey, MD.. He was not by
experience and training, then, a liver transplant
surgeon. Whether for that reason, or others, David
had a ghastly time after surgery, mainly with bile
leaks which caused infections, until Dr. Thomas
Broughan rerouted the bile ducts. Before that
definitive surgery, he had two life threatening
infections, other less serious ones and had to have
stents placed every two months to drain sub-hepatic
fluids. He recalls infections every week from bile
leaks on and off for five months. After transplant he
lost about eighty pounds; he refused to eat. At this
point in his history, Dr. Natalie Murray was the
hepatologist in charge at Methodist Hospital, and had
enjoined David's wife, Janet, to be her nurse
coordinator for the liver transplant program. Janet
had been practicing in the emergency room
previously, and it was there that she had met the
fireman who was to become her husband. Between
the two of them, Natalie and Janet, and with David's
own operative will power, he started eating again
and began to improve.

David has come through very well, and
attributes his healing to the central role which mind

control and positive attitude played. Actually, he attributes his currently healthy, happy state of being to his wife, but for his part, he says that he did a lot of reading about maintaining a positive attitude and tried to practice what he preached. He has had his time of depression and mood swings. About a year ago he felt that at 47 he was wasting his life, just sitting around. Even working on his beloved sail boat was not enough. After his initial commitment to live, because of Janet, -- in his words -- "After putting her through all this, I wasn't going to just sit here and die on her," and so he determined to eat. Later, he watched her go off to work while he, the designated main bread winner, just sat around. So he determined to go back to school and is studying to be a surgical technician and perhaps, down the line, a registered nurse. Meanwhile, David participates with very good reason, in Janet's preoccupation with donor awareness, with active volunteerism in different forums of transplant advocacy. Believe me, they make some kind of team.

More up front and personal, David talked about his diminished libido. After transplant he felt no sexual desire, just apathy. Two years after transplant, he said that he could care less, but believes a lot was psychological, and perhaps the

"Other Voices, Other Rooms"

result of medication. It is the factor of medication
which I asked Dr. Murray about. David takes both
Calan for blood pressure and Prozac for depression.
With regard to his psyche and mental adjustment,
he wisely commented that he can't psyche himself
up to relax, or cut himself off from intimacy, and
then try it, and fail, and then fail to try again. He
and Janet can talk though, and he says that now
things are getting better. In the usual male manner,
he said that men won't talk to each other about
sexual dysfunction and he doesn't want to talk to a
psychiatrist who doesn't know him. Fortunately for
David, his wife, long-suffering though human as she
is, is a nurse, and knows a little bit about all these
symptoms.

In response to my queries about post-
transplant medications and decreased sexual drive
or impotency, Dr. Murray discounted the primacy of
drugs as the cause of the problems. According to
Natalie, (and the following is transcribed almost
word for word):

What patients don't appreciate is that
the intense process of liver disease and
some of the insults that led to the liver
disease, set them up for diminished libido,

and in men, impotence. There is in men a higher expectation of performance, and more anxiety associated with it. Prior to transplant, there are a lot of things that insult the body of the cirrhotic that ends up leading to sexual dysfunction.

Sexual function is mediated by a hormonal access that begins in the brain with the part that controls autonomic and hormonal functions, specifically in the hypothalamus, which sends messages to the pituitary gland -- sends out all the factors that support the gonads, which in turn provide hormones which support both function and libido. Excess intake of alcohol, long term cirrhosis and encephalopathy, hemachromatosis all upset this access at varying points. Some of this is reversed at transplant; some of it is not.

Feeling horrible diminishes sex drive; but there is a real psychological problem as well. Aldactone (a diuretic) before transplant affects sexual function in men. It can cause impotence. Post-operatively, drugs may impact sexual function. Overall, steroids don't have so much effect.

116

"Other Voices, Other Rooms"

Hypertension drugs have the potential
of causing impotence. Depression can cause
impotence, so can anti-depressant drugs.
Sometimes other systemic problems
which persist preclude the physician's
flexibility in changing to drugs with less
potent effects.

Natalie believes too in the role of the psyche
and the emotions. She has observed that those who
feel sorry for themselves, who assume the victim
role, or remain in a dependent mode, do less well in
all of their energies including their sexual activity.
As with most illnesses and most invasive
treatments, afterwards doing more, exercising,
getting back to work, resuming a normal life style,
allows one to do even more. Exercise is invaluable
in the healing process, good for emotional well-being
as well as helpful in lowering blood pressure and
cholesterol levels. Libido? It only stands to reason
that feeling healthy, achieving a sense of well being
and control contributes to a kind of natural
aphrodisiac, not available at health aids stores.

117

I'm Glad You're Not Dead

MARCIE: WAITING/IMPROVING

Marcie announced at the support group at her
first meeting that she was an alcoholic. She was, by
this time, sober for a year, used to the candor of AA
meetings. I was not present at this enjoinder, but I
understand that she felt awkward at her admission,
since it was met with silence, and not with the
expected reply. She drank for fifteen years and was
diagnosed with a fatty liver nine years ago. It had
since progressed to cirrhosis. After the first
diagnosis she couldn't stay sober. She would stop
drinking after she began having bleeds, then feel
well, and begin drinking again. She experienced
perhaps a month of sobriety between bleeds. One
hemorrhage she remembers most vividly occurred
during her drive from New Jersey to Texas. She had
lost her job, a crisis which started her drinking
again, and intended to move to Texas to be near her
brother. She hemorrhaged on the way, but merely
rested overnight at a motel and kept going the next
day.

She continued drinking in her new location.
She attributes the addiction to a psychological
dependency and her own insecurities. She believes
now that she had hoped she would die, a
disappointment to everyone, including herself. Her

"Other Voices, Other Rooms"

last bleed precipitated a coma that lasted almost a month. She awoke, miraculously, without mental impairment, determined to assume responsibility for herself. With a real humility and an incredible willingness, sober now for more than a year, she waits for definitive improvement, or, if it becomes necessary, transplant.

JUDY: WAITING

Judy has been waiting for a liver for almost three years. Thirty months ago she was told that her Hepatitis C had progressed to end stage liver disease. Her history extends back to the mid-seventies when she contracted what was then recognized as non A, non B hepatitis from her former husband, a drug addict.

The long wait has taken its toll on her sensibilities and her dignity. She suffers intensely from extreme ascites and encephalopathy. She says that sometimes she loses days now; she is disoriented, loses control over little things. She can't dial the phone, use the remote control, read or write, do simple math, on especially bad days. The encephalopathy comes and goes, and when it is present it is as if there is a mist over everything. It is like being in a fog. Sometimes her speech is affected; she can't fill out simple forms. She lives

I'm Glad You're Not Dead

with fatigue, dizziness, a ringing in her ears,
forgetful and knowing it. She will live like this until
a suitable organ is found that matches her rare
blood type, or until it is too late.

These folk, this fair field of folk, to echo Piers
Plowman, represent the many, the pre and post
transplant patients. They are my friends and I love
them. They have come into my life in an
unexpected, unsought way. There is a bond among
us which we share with no one else in our lives. We
share this bond also with the five thousand people
awaiting liver transplant each day in this country
and with the six who die each day waiting.

Chapter Eight
"American Graffiti"

We Americans are a peculiar lot. We drive
ourselves as our Puritan founding forebearers
would have wished, regardless of our race or
religion, and so are extremely productive and
fittingly rigid in our work ethic. We are then
proportionately excessive in other arenas of life.
We eat too much, drink too much, sit too much, and
some of us indulge in even more destructive habits
and lifestyle choices. We seem incabable of
moderation and/or balance. One might almost say
that we are prone, or propelled, to liver disease.
Now we have managed to pollute our air, and so can
run around ingesting, or breathing , toxins to our
hearts' discontent.

When we "reform" we are apt to be excessive in
our reformation. Dr. Murray remarked on people
who decide they want to live a healthy life and then

embrace unproven and even dangerous practices under the guise of natural or folk health practices:

A lot that gets packaged and sold, advertised as good and natural, can be dangerous to persons with a particular problem or to people in general when they overdo. Americans seem to think that a lot is better than a little.

Just because a recommended dosage or intake is presented--still people ignore the label, or overdo; many substances come with no recommendation at all. Excess Vitamin A can cause cirrhosis and liver failure, and yet huge doses are available in health food stores. People receive no warning. Teas such as gensing and chaparral have caused hepatic necrosis and auto-liver failure. Patients have required transplantation for that. What worries me is when patients learn they have liver disease and start taking things. Many substances untested in normals have been around for years without ill effect. The same substances may harm patients with significant liver disease. The same is true of standard medications.

Dr. Murray proclaimed her concern over the great American quest for either self-destruction or health in the extreme. We embrace the diet craze;

"American Graffiti"

we visit third world countries without vaccinations,
eat and drink in our travels indiscriminately. Back
to nature people ingest wild mushrooms and are
poisoned. Liver failure results. Tatoos run right
after IV drugs as a source for Hepatitis C contracted
by sub-cutaneous exposure. Currently rock stars
glamorize tatoos, and young people, "got to have
'em," while young people from the past are turning
up with Hepatitis from their college drug
experimentation days.

As a people, our lifestyle choices leave a lot to
be desired. Some vary by region. Dr. Thomas
Broughan, in interview, commented on the contrast,
and his shock, between his "carriage trade" at the
Cleveland Clinic, and his current practice in Texas at
UTMB, a medical center known as an indigent
hospital:

> When I came here [Texas], I came
> from a lovely, fashionable practice at
> the Cleveland Clinic, and I came here
> where things weren't so pretty. I
> thought that all I needed to do was
> throw money at these patients, and
> everything would turn out all right,
> and I found that for psychosocial
> reasons, even if patients are afforded

123

I'm Glad You're Not Dead

what I think is the very best in health
care, some of them either don't know how,
or don't want to seize the opportunity.
They get sick and don't call,don't come in,
wait until it's too late, continue the same
habits that rob them of any improved
health. I realized that just because I
could reach in and provide them with
health care that they had never had
access to, had never been able to afford. . .
I was amazed; I was flabergasted that
people rejected it, didn't follow it, didn't
take advantage of it. I didn't think
anybody would do that. Some people have
it set in their minds that their health isn't
a priority, and it is not important to take
care of oneself. They go on smoking,
drinking, engage in other dangerous
behavior. Geography, lower socio-
economic profiles contribute to these
attitudes and lifestyles. The South,
perhaps Texas in particular, is not as
health conscious as other parts of the
country. Even well to do people don't
seem to take good care of themselves.
People here seem to really live hard and
not take care of themselves. I notice this

"American Graffiti"

with both recipients and donors.

   I have already written of the fatty liver
syndrome, characteristic of some Americans,
certainly of those who consume too much alcohol
and/or fatty foods. These constitute many of the
potential donors who are rejected by selective
surgeons. Some livers are not rejected and should
be, and thereby contribute to a low graft survival
rate, causing patient death or retransplantation. I
am once again grateful for my conscientious surgeon
who, with administrators metaphorically breathing
down his neck, rejected three fatty livers, organs of
women all about fifty, before transplanting me. We
cannot hope, perversely, that our young people, out
of their recklessness, or violence, or untimely
deaths, be our organ banks. Can we ever count on
our citizens to love their bodies, to care for their
gift?
   Statistics of young, sometimes very young
people who consume alcohol regularly and in
careless quantity alarm the American public. Their
elders, ignorant themselves of what might be ahead,
offer no information and no control. A liver is a
terrible organ to waste. Sexual promiscuity may

also be the source of liver disease. Hepatitis B and probably C may be transmitted by bodily fluids.

Liver transplantation, now a technical possibility, is exhorbitantly costly. Health care economics cannot sustain unlimited transplant surgeries. Unlike heart and lung disease, however, there are no surgeon general warnings issued to the population to alert them to prevention or avoidance in the matter of liver disease. The only destruction signalled by social advertising has to do with psychosocial outcomes: abuse of alcohol leads to domestic violence, dysfunctional families, highway accidents. If cirrhosis is mentioned, it sounds like something one might suffer from a little. Being a little cirrhotic is like being a little pregnant. Its product is not life, however, but death in all too many cases. The progression of the disease, outlined in these chapters, is devastating. No pleasurable entertainments, or careless behaviors are worth the ghastly human suffering.

If people can be "scared straight" in our society as the result of visits to prisons, then I suggest similar therapy for those who make certain lifestyle choices while they can still change. Let them visit with those who are awaiting liver transplant as a result of their own behavior patterns, or visit an ER while a cirrhotic is on the table bleeding from every

orifice, or talk with a dying pre or post transplant
patient whose body was too ravaged by the disease
and by certain behaviors to withstand the "cure."
Our "partying" might change drastically.

Chapter Nine
"To Arrive Where We Started"

I returned to my ocean view, my homeplace, in far better health than I had left it. I had reached and o'er leapt the apex of my adventure. Now all that remained was to heal and gain strength. I returned with a certain timidity. I wasn't taking any risks with diet, and I was rigidly cautious about medication. The ordeal of transplant is so enormous that, while one is subject to a lot of programing by health care personnel before discharge, most of the brainwashing having to do with the medication and other orders come from within. I cannot imagine anyone going through all this grief, only to be careless afterwards, chancing rejection episodes, or infection, by personal laxity. I knew to avoid even the dearest people if they approached me with any contagion, even an old cold, and not to be in the same room for awhile yet with fresh flowers or

plants because of their exposure to pesticides and
other toxins.

The day of discharge, in the midst of my
preening, and while waiting for hospital bureaucracy
to catch up with itself, I determined that I badly
needed a haircut. I had no idea when I could visit
my regular stylist again, so I walked down, dressed
of course, to the hospital salon. I was well into the
haircut when I noticed a man-eating plant
practically draped over my shoulder. It was clear
that I was not yet into good habits of scoping out a
room for danger zones. Suddenly, over the other
shoulder loomed Natalie, gleefully presiding with a
kind of "I caught you" leer, and proclaiming that I
made it awfully difficult to make rounds. She had
really come on an official good-bye. We walked
together back to the ward like two veterans of the
same war, a war which, so far, we had won.

I've gotten off with relative ease, at least so
far. I am now almost nine months beyond
transplant surgery. At anytime, for the rest of my
life, any infection is dangerous because of my drug
regime which is deliberately imposed in order to
suppress my immune system. An ordinary illness,
relatively benign for a healthy person, could become
virulent for the immune suppressed person. So, of
course, could toxic substances and foods. I'll never

eat raw fish again, and I'll always be careful about drinking water. I will be a consistent consumer of "Veggie Wash," and never again steal an unwashed grape from a supermarket display. I'll never drink alcohol again. I am still careful about kisses. The problem with good friends, who want to plant one on me, is that they may think at the time that they are infection free, but come down with a cold or flu the next day. Meanwhile, I have been exposed. I caught two colds this past winter, shortly after discharge, this way. I did not, fortunately, run a fever with either, so there was no real threat. I was miserable because, unlike my fellow sufferers, I couldn't pop aspirin or antihistimines.

All of the anti-rejection, immunesuppressant drugs on the market have unpleasant side affects which manifest in different ways with different people. They can be adjusted by doctors, or substituted for by other anti-immune drugs with the same effect but never eliminated, lest the body reject the new organ. I still both marvel and chafe at the physiological fact that with my new, 26 year old liver, I could be as healthy as a horse, were it not that every day I pump prednisone and cyclosporine into my system to lower its ability to fight off infection, and foreign bodies. This is some kind of irony.

I'm Glad You're Not Dead

Over time, however, as the dosage is reduced, I
will build up, white cell count included, something of
my own immune system again, never what it could
be without drug therapy, but better and better, the
farther from surgery and the lower the dosage.

Often, after surgery the patient's blood
pressure is consistently high. Mine was, and is now
normal. I did not have to take any blood pressure
medicine, nor any medication for depression, most
commonly prozac. These meds, too, have their
unwelcome side effects. Cyclosporine almost always
raises choloesterol and triglycerides in the patient.
My numbers are too high, in spite of my close
monitoring of fat and sodium in my diet. I am
hopeful that as the cyclosporine levels decrease, so
will the cholosterol and tryglicerides. There is a
direct correlation. In just the last two months I
have experienced tolerable but unwelcome
perepheral neuropathy in my hands and feet, and
significant insomnia. These indicators, too, are
correlative with a still high daily dose of
cyclosporine. In the case of a transplant patient,
however, it is not a matter of the cure being worse
than the disease. Without these immune
suppressent drugs, still so new to modern medicine,
there could be no transplant survivors, whatever

the organ involved. I'll take the side effects, forever, if necessary.

Perhaps because they are sometimes so difficult, transplant physicians and personnel worry most after surgery about patients not taking their medications. In Janet's own words:

> My biggest worry is that on down the line they'll get lax, listen to other people's advice, stop taking their meds. First, I've thought well, maybe they just don't understand. We have a lawyer who's had her liver eight years and has just decided that she doesn't like what the medicine is doing to her -- she's taking herbs. That's always my fear, that they'll listen to someone, that a kidney transplant patient will tell a heart or liver transplant that "I don't take that much predisone," and one will think, hey, if they don't, why should I?

The results could be deadly. I am taking, however, fewer medications than I was before surgery. I honestly feel healthy: my energy level is probably higher than most people my age. I have, however, had fewer post-transplant problems than others whom I know. I cannot account for my condition

I'm Glad You're Not Dead

except for the efficacy of my mental and emotional
state before and after surgery, and my relative
physical well being. My damaged liver had not yet
ravaged my other organs. The new liver was indeed
a good match even down to the fit of the hepatic
artery. Nor have I had problems with bile duct
leakage. Before surgery, too, aspects of my profile
were atypical. My bleeds, for example, were not
from ruptured varices (veins that burst in the lower
end of the esophagus), and I was very careful with
nutrition. I have mentioned the role which prayer
played in my recovery. There are too many sources
for me to list. Many of them emanated from my
Mother who is always a kind of prayer Chairwoman.
She solicited the spiritual efforts of all those around
her, most, but not all, known to me. My family
sustained me, too. My brother, Dan, was unusually
solicitous. Dan's a good guy, but like most brothers
sometimes emotionally inaccessible, to his credit, not
this time. He was very present. My sister Kathy,
the only seamstress in our family, sent endless
arrays of one-size fits all lounge garments, very
welcome in this disease, for the sick person bounces
around in sizes because of variable fluid retention.
My father was, as always, the silent strong one in
the background, supporting and loving, from his
position, so long now pronounced, of mainstay. And

"To Arrive Where We Started"

Ann. What can I say? I couldn't have made it without her.

So many friends held me up. I came home to celebration, shortly before Thanksgiving. It was that and more! How could it not have been. This year I didn't cook, but I could have, and I succeeded in meddling mightily. The night before Thanksgiving Ann and I went to a department store and bought a new couch -- a fine one in Italian leather. There were not many people out shopping the evening before Thanksgiving, so my exposure was minimal. Even so, I held my breath around small children and placed a Kleenex between my hand and the escalator rail. These are the habits which diminish as life goes on in an active and normal way. If there is no intermittent reaction to ordinary protocol, then the transplant patient falls pretty easily into casual modes of behavior. I will admit that my caution level has lowered throughout the last several months. It has not reached dangerous levels because I do not take chances. I am comfortable but not complacent with the stability of my health.

I encountered more challenge on the emotional than the physical level during the early days. After Thanksgiving and through Christmas, I sustained a period of peace and gratitude, and a time of being touched, sentimentally, by almost anything of a tender nature. I cried easily, or at least got watery. I had some difficulty reconciling my immense good fortune, my gift of life, with a very humble self-concept. I wrestled with unworthiness, but at this point, I gave in to acceptance. I was at peace. I sometimes consciously entered into peace.

Christmas affirmed it. My immediate local family and I planned a feast in every meaning of the word. We would dress up, really dress up -- jewels and all, go out to eat in a place with a fitting ambience, elegant and expensive, but not loud and crowded, tending to the hushed undertones of our communal spirits, and then go to Midnight Mass. It seemed more than appropriate that I extend my thanksgiving to the altar of the Lord, but I have a real problem with most priests' sermons, and I am, to put it mildly, disenchanted with the patriarchal nature of the Church. Nevertheless, participation in the Eucharist was more than incumbent on me this Christmas. I decided that we, Ann, Margaret, Linda and I should not expect a good homily (sermon) and just look around the city for a better than average choir. We decided on an Afro-American Church, the only one in small town Galveston. They would surely have, in spite of their Catholic persuasion, joyful, maybe even gospel music. We were almost right, except that, sure enough, the emotional and

136

ritual constraints of the Catholic Church impacted on the spontaneity of the choir and congregation more than a little. Still not entirely used to avoidance of crowds, and only two months beyond surgery, I had forgotten that Catholics of whatever race, or state of alienation, attend Mass on Easter, Christmas and Mother's Day. The church was so packed that, as with an Italian crowd, one could pick up both feet and still be "standing." Since it was winter, coughing, sneezing, rasping surrounded me. My nervous Nellies started gesturing for me to leave. I dug in. Ann told me to hold a tissue in front of my face. I thought great -- here are we, the only few white faces in an all black church, and she wants me to stand here holding my nose. No deal. In spite of these agitations, Mass was, for me, a blessed event, and all of Christmas memorable. I did not catch a cold as the result of my piety. That was left for a friend of mine to impart at a New Year's Eve party.

Subsequent to this season of peace and joy, and natural highs, I began to feel other, conflicting emotions, some guilt, some confusion, built around the circumstances of my undeserved good fortune.

I think every transplant patient must go through this anguish. Like victims of other attacks, I blamed myself for the disease. I had neglected my health for all of my adult life, going without regular

check-ups, ignoring symptoms, careless about
exposure and excess. I went through a prolonged
period of guilt in which I apologized ad nauseum to
those whom my illness had most affected. I just felt
so rotten that I had put loved ones through the
agony of anguishing over me, waiting with me, like
me, putting their lives on hold. And then I felt
confused, simultaneously, at the freely bestowed gift
of life. I cried easily when I faced my guilt/gift
conundrum. Well, I cried easily anyway -- mood
swings attend prednisone drug therapy. A young
man, Ruben, transplanted about the same time as I,
complained of the inexplicable onset of rage. I just
turned on the faucet. So now part of my charm
consisted in blubbering while I either castigated
myself or exulted in each day's beauty and my
future hope.

All of the emotional highs and lows plane out,
too. I left the hospital on a 20 milligrams per day
prednisone schedule. I now take 10 milligrams daily.
I am aiming at five, then none, down the road. This
medication adjustment, and my own attempts at
getting a grip, have stabilized my mood swings. On
the one hand, I have decided that whatever my role
in my illness, I have definitely suffered enough, and
on the other hand, I have held to the belief that life
is a gift.

"To Arrive Where We Started"

I also believe it to be a responsibility. All of my life I have heard it echoed that when much is given, much is, conversely, expected. I have been given, in middle age, a new beginning. I have a grave responsibility to use it well, for benefit, while I give myself permission to enjoy it.

I undertook to write this book for two reasons: to put into easy availability a volume which might become a kind of road map and source of information for those who need it -- a compendium of information with a personal frame narrative. I did not have one, and found, instead, disparate and fragmented, cryptic pieces of information. My second reason for writing this "manual" is to extend an earnest, desperate call for organ donation.

I have known people who died waiting for an organ. I waited for fifteen months after being listed in the system. My blood type is O positive, not uncommon. I talk with people, see them, see them declining every month at clinic or support group meetings. I visit them on the ward when they are "in" for an infection or bleed, or pleural effusions. Each time, their eyes are less bright, their smiles more tentative. In direct proportion their wives, husbands, mothers are more determined, staving off by will, reflected in daring eyes, a dark fate. They seem to say: "Hold it off, hold it off, yet a little longer."

Against this human background, I have great difficulty understanding objections to organ donation. I know that many are sincere, engendered by religious or ethnic consideration, but even for this population I urge them to consult their leaders, lest they have misconstrued their teachings, or can even effect a change in their not so well founded attitudes. For those who worry that their donation may affect their end time health care, I beg them to inquire of appropriate persons, and satisfy themselves in this regard. Organ donation is such a simple matter; organ reception so inordinately difficult.

Once again my narrative was interrupted, this time by a simple, very American, very normal demand. On August 14, 1995, my birthday, less than ten months after surgery, I returned to work. I am now, at this writing, mid-way through an academic semester, very much integrated into my teaching schedule and environment, and feeling, physically, like I was never transplanted. My energy level and over-all well being probably provided me with the opportunity to resume work earlier, but my profession did not. I live my life by semesters, and

"To Arrive Where We Started"

so had to wait for the fall to roll around, lest I transplant some substitute in my classes.

I have had little trouble adjusting to campus life. I still see all the world with new vision, however, and this soul-sight occasionally presents me with mind-stopping insights and quick heaves of thanksgiving. I am a different person following in my own footsteps around campus, just a little out of focus, waiting for the new me to catch up with the old one, or vice versa, in a kind of double vision, not yet quite integrated. I'll let you know when I conjoin.

Meanwhile, I'll drop you off from this journey I started you on. I don't know if I've been a Vergil or a Beatrice to your Dante out there. I pray that because of this book, you have it less hard, less in ignorance and in doubt. There is definitely full life after transplant. I began this last chapter with a quotation from T. S. Eliot's "Little Gidding." In context it reads:

> We shall not cease from exploration
> And the end of all our exploring
> Will be to arrive where we started
> And know the place for the first time.

I'm Glad You're Not Dead

I know, for the fullest time, my home, my family, my friends and the effulgent, eternal gift of life.

October 24, 1995. One year after transplant.

GLOSSARY

a

abdominal drain - a plastic tube that allows blood, serum, and bile to exit the peritoneal cavity without difficulty.

ADL - activities of daily living

Alpha-fetoprotein (AFP) - a protein produced in the liver and gastrointestinal tract of adults having hepatitis or cirrhosis.

AMA - Anti-mitrocuondrial antibody (see ANA).

ammonia - a byproduct of protein metabolism normally produced in the body; a malfunctioning liver inhibits the processing of ammonia and its accompanying compounds. These toxins build up, causing encephalopathy, or in extreme cases, coma.

ANA - Anti-nuclear antibody -- evidence that the body has been fooled and is attacking itself, including the liver, in autoimmune disease.

angiogram - a process by which blood vessels can be x-rayed in order to determine their normal/abnormal arrangement and potency.

ascites - water retention in the abdominal area; the kidneys become confused and do not excrete the sodium and water that they should.

b

bile duct - a duct or tube leading from the liver to the gallbladder and small intestine. Bile is formed from broken-down, old red blood cells and functions as a detergent in the absorption of fat from one's diet.

bile duct leakage - following transplant, bile duct attached to the transplanted organ which were attached to existing duct of the recipient may leak prior to healing. These leaks may require remedial surgery.

biliary flow - the flow of bile in the ducts.

biopsy - a method by which the liver is "sampled"
with a needle; the needle collects liver tissue at
varying depths, which can then be analyzed.

bypass - in liver transplant surgery, a procedure
performed in order to return blood from the
lower half of the body to the heart.

C

cardiology - the study of the heart.

catheter - a tube placed in the bladder to drain
urine.

cauterize - a process of stopping tissue from
bleeding through the use of heat or chemicals
(also, see endoscopy).

CBC - a test which measures the number of white
and red cells.

central line - a reliable and quick-access IV, usually
inserted in the neck that extends into the major
veins of the chest.

cholangiogram - a test to determine the potency and
integrity of the bile ducts.

cholesterol - made by the liver particularly from
saturated fats.

cirrhotic - scarred tissue; a cirrhotic liver looks as if there were a string of pearls pushing up through the flesh.

clostridium difficile - a germ that makes a toxin in the colon that can overgrow and cause diarrhea.

coagulase negative staph - an increasingly common infection-causing germ.

comatose - a state of unconsciousness.

compis mentis - being mentally competent.

cryoprecipitate - a concentrate of blood clotting components that is separated from units of donated blood.

cryptogenic - hidden origin; medical jargon for, "we don't know."

cryptogenic cirrhosis - scarring of the liver, the cause of which is unknown.

CT scan - also called CAT (Computerized Axial Tomographic) scan. This technique uses a combination of computer and x-ray which, in combination, will provide a cross-sectional image of the tissue or body being examined.

cyclosporine - an immunosuppressant drug used to prevent the body from rejecting the new organ, otherwise interpreted by the body as a foreign object which should be attacked. This drug threatens serious side effects, but it is usually essential to life following transplant (also, see predisone).

d

diuretics - medication prescribed for water retention; excess fluids are expelled through the kidneys.

dopamine - used to assist the body in renal and blood pressure functions. It is a vasoconstrictor naturally produced by the brain but can be injected through an IV for patients who need blood pressure support. At low doses, it can help the kidneys produce urine.

e

ECG - Also called EKG. See electrocardiogram.

echocardiogram - a technique used to obtain an image of the heart through the use of sound waves.

EKG - Also called ECG. See electrocardiogram.

eletrocardiogram - a tracing which shows the electrical conductivity of the heart.

encephalopathy - mental confusion due to toxins in the bloodstream..

endoscopy - a tube with a light and video camera which is inserted through the mouth and intestines in order to visually diagnose. This procedure is common in the case of suspected ruptured varices. Tissue can be cauterized or injected during this procedure when necessary.

endotracheal tube - a tube placed in the wind pipe (usually through the mouth) and attached to a ventilator to assist the patient with breathing.

enterococcus - a germ that causes infection and can be problematic to eliminate.

enzyme levels - the liver contains many enzymes, some of which can be tested in the blood to try to determine the relative health of the liver.

extrahepatic malignancy - cancer outside the liver.

f

fatty liver - In appearance, it is large, smooth and
    pale, i.e., it is fat. About 25% of the population
    has a fatty liver, and it is a common response by
    the liver when there is trauma/injury.
febrile - having a fever.
fresh frozen plasma - clotting factors derived from
    the blood used to treat bleeding.

g

gastroenterologist - a physician who has a broad
    specialization in the digestive system, from the
    mouth to the anus, including the stomach, liver,
    intestines, kidneys, pancreas, and gallbladder.
globulin - produced by the liver; gamma globulins or
    immunoglobulins are antibodies which are
    produced in the blood stream following liver

transplant. They can fight infection and/or cause rejection.

graft - an organ transplant.

gram positive cocci - germs which cause infection and include coagulase negative staphylococcus and enterococcus.

GTT - Glucose Tolerance Test - helps to determine if an individual has diabetes.

h

harvest - the removal of a donor organ for the purpose of transplantation.

Health Panel - multiple blood tests that are ordered together as a group (for example: tests for the amount of cholesterol or liver enzymes).

hematocrit - a test to determine how many blood cells are contained in a given volumn of blood.

hemochromatosis - abnormal processing and storage of iron by the body.

hemodynamic instability - the state of having widely variable blood pressure and pulse. It can be found in a number of situations characterized by lack of blood and/or compromised heart function.

hemoglobin - the element in your blood which
carries and deposits oxygen to the rest of your
body.

hemorrhoids - swollen tissue which extends outside
the anal opening.

hepatic - anything related to the liver.

hepatic artery - the blood vessel which carries
freshly oxygenated blood to the liver.

hepatobiliary surgeon - hepatic refers to the liver;
biliary refers to bile, i.e., the liquid secreted by
the liver through ducts. A hepatobiliary
surgeon, then, is one who focuses on surgical
diseases of the liver, gallbladder, and bile ducts.

hepatic pathology - a general term relating to all
disorders of the liver.

hepatitis antibodies - an indicator that one has been
previously exposed to hepatitis. These
antibodies can be identified through a blood test.

hepatitis - inflammation of the liver coupled with
cell damage. The three most common types of
veral hepatitis: A, B, and C (previously known
as non-A, non-B).

hepatologist - a physician who has specialized in the
study of the liver and its diseases.

herniated navel - the protrusion of the intestine or
fluid through the abdominal wall near the navel.

HMO - Health Maintenance Organization

hydration - introducing/maintaining water into the
body, in this case, through an IV.

i, j, k

immunosuppression - prohibiting the body's
immune system from attacking the new organ.
Immunosuppression is achieved through drugs
immediately following transplant and continued
throughout the recipient's life.

immunosuppression drugs - drugs which reduce the
activity of the body's immune system.
Cyclosporine and prednisone are most common
although research promises alternatives in the
future.

internalist - a physician who has specialized in
diseases affecting internal organs.

intraoperatively - within an operation

Iron Studies - blood tests by which the level of iron
in one's system can be determined. Too much
iron in the body can cause cirrhosis of the liver.

l

lactulose - a drug which softens the feces, acts as a laxative and helps to eliminate toxins from being absorbed from the colon into the bloodstream.

laparoscopy - insertion of a scope into the abdomen through a stab wound to view the internal organs.

laparotomy - An operation involving opening the abdominal cavity which enables the physician to view the liver .

Lasix - a diuretic that helps the kidneys to make urine.

m, n

nasogastric tube - a tube inserted through the nose and into the stomach in order to drain secretions and air.

NPO - Non per os , i.e., nothing by mouth.

O

Organ Procurement Organization (OPO) - a regionally governed center which facilitates organ distribution in a given area; (also see UNOS).
orthotopic liver transplant - the surgery necessary to perform the transplant. The prefix "ortho" means normal, or straight. Orthotopic, then, refers to placing the new liver exactly where the old one was.

p, q

paracentesis - a process to remove/withdraw excess fluid from the periotoneal cavity using a needle. It is a quick and relatively easy process and only a local anesthetic is necessary.
peripheral neuropathy - an inflamation of the nerves resulting in numbness, tingling, or pain in the extemities.
perioperative period - around the time of surgery.
platelets - an element of the blood which causes clotting.

pleural effusion - the collection of fluid around the lungs.

portal hypertension - this refers to increased pressure in the veins around the liver and intestines. A scarred, cirrhotic liver resists the normal flow of venous blood from the intestines through it. This resistence causes increased pressure in these veins and more veins (varices in the esophogus and stomach) open up to try to handle this increased pressure. This condition is directly related to an enlarged spleen and ascites.

prednisone - a steroid used after transplant to prevent rejection of the new organ. Like cyclosporine, this is a nasty drug with possible serious side effects, but it is essential to life for the transplant recipient.

prozac - a medication prescribed for depression.

PT- Prothrombin time; a test for coagulation time.

r

red blood cells - that element of one's blood which absorbs oxygen and delivers/releases it to the body tissue.

rejection - when the body recognizes the new organ as foreign and attacks. Immediately following transplant, most recipients go through mild rejection. A rule of thumb is to expect rejection on about the seventh day following surgery. One should expect mild rejection It is managed with modification in medications.

renal - anything referring to the kidney.

ruptured varices - veins that burst in the lower esophagus.

S

septic - the state of having a serious infection. If one is "septic" or has "sepsis," one should expect some degree of encephalopathy.

SICU - Surgical Intensive Care Unit

staph infection - bacteria present in membranes. There are good bacteria, bad bacteria. The high doses of antibiotics required of a recent transplant patient will kill some bacteria and allow others to grow; thus, a yeast infection is common among female recipients.

subhepatic fluid - blood and/or serum collected under the liver.

systemic infection - an infection which is found throughout the entire system. Synonymous with sepsis (see Septic).

t

T-tube - a tube placed in the bile duct in order to drain bile into a small pouch outside the body. It is shaped like a "T" with the tail of the "T" visible from the outside of the body. The top of the "T" is positioned in the bile duct.

tracheostomy - (also referred to as "trache") - a tube inserted through the mouth in order to maintain an adequate airway. It is usually removed two or three days after surgery.

triglycerides - fat in the bloodstream.

u

ultrasound - a method of diagnosing a liver condition using sound waves.

UNOS - See United Network for Organ Sharing.

United Network for Organ Sharing (UNOS) - a non
   profit, federally funded, private organization
   which accounts for organs and their distribution
   throughout the country. This "mother
   company" maintains the national data base,
   which in turn, is accessed by OPO's.

V, W, X, y, Z

Vancomycin - an antibiotic used to treat staph
   infections.

varices - enlarged veins (similar to varicose veins),
   which develop in the lower esophagus and
   stomach. They can also present as hemorrhoids.

viral hepatitis - Hepatis can be spread through a
   virus. Types A, B, and C are spread
   differently; any viral hepatitis attacks the liver
   (see Hepatic). Hepatitis is not always viral. For
   instance, it can be caused by drugs, or it can be
   autoimmune in origin.